Persistent Fat and How to Lose It

By the same authors:

Cured to Death: the Effects of Prescription Drugs
The Long-Life Heart: How to Avoid Heart Disease and Live a
Longer Life

Persistent Fat and How to Lose It

ARABELLA MELVILLE and
COLIN JOHNSON

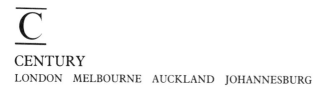

CENTURY
LONDON MELBOURNE AUCKLAND JOHANNESBURG

First published in 1986 by Century Hutchinson Ltd,
Brookmount House, 62–65 Chandos Place, Covent Garden,
London WC2N 4NW

Century Hutchinson Publishing Group (Australia) Pty Ltd
16–22 Church Street, Hawthorn, Melbourne, Victoria 3122

Century Hutchinson Group (NZ) Ltd
32–34 View Road, PO Box 40-086, Glenfield, Auckland 10

Century Hutchinson Group (SA) Pty Ltd
PO Box 337, Bergvlei 2012, South Africa

Set in Plantin

British Library Cataloguing in Publication Data

Melville, Arabella
  Persistent fat and how to lose it : the safe
  guide to permanent weight loss.
  1. Obesity——Treatment
  I. Title   II. Johnson, Colin, *1939–*
  616.3'9806   RC628

  ISBN 0-7126-1142-8

Printed in Great Britain by
St Edmundsbury Press, Bury St Edmunds, Suffolk

For Inge

Acknowledgements

Many people have helped us with this book. We cannot name those in official positions who gave off-the-record information, but we nevertheless thank them. We are also grateful to those Life Profile clients whose experiences we have drawn upon to develop the theory and illustrate this text.

Special thanks are due to Dr John Watts, who shared with us a wealth of information and expertise and contributed to discussions on the PFR phenomenon. Dr Chris Upton, Professor Brian Kettering and Peter Bunyard each gave generously of time and knowledge.

We are grateful to our publishers, Century Hutchinson, for their patience and enthusiasm.

Finally, we would like to acknowledge the persistence and encouragement of our agent, David Grossman, throughout the conception, gestation and birth of this book.

Contents

CHAPTER 1

What This Book Will Do For You

This book is not for everyone. It is written for those who seriously wish to lose persistent fat. Its aim is to explain the cause of what we call the Persistent Fat Retention or PFR Syndrome and to put you in charge of your body so that you can control the amount of fat you carry. Although dietary change is involved, this is not a diet book. If you are one of those unfortunate people who, for whatever psychological reason, need to diet continually without achieving anything positive, this book is not for you.

Before going any further you should ask yourself the following questions:

Do I really want to have a slim and attractive body?

Can I cope with being in control of my body?

Am I absolutely sure I am not hiding behind fat and failure?

If you can say an emphatic 'Yes!' to any two of these questions, then reading this book will help you in the following ways.

It will show you how to lose persistent fat. By this we mean not only ordinary body fat, but also cellulite and that unhealthy watery flab, those unwanted tissues which resist all the reducing methods you may have previously tried. It may also explain problems of clinical obesity, both in adults and children. It will teach you how to maintain your body at your desired weight for the rest of your life, with methods which are progressive, natural and entirely safe. It will enhance your looks because it will improve that essential foundation of all beauty, inner health. It will introduce you to holistic concepts of living. And once you have lost your persistent weight, it will teach you how to achieve the sort of body shape you desire.

Finally, it will explain why many of the other methods of weight loss you may have tried have failed to achieve permanent results, and why many of them may actually damage your health and even contribute to your unwanted fat problem.

For some time we have been successfully helping a wide range of people with this problem. It is this experience which makes us sure that we are not making the sort of extravagant claims which you will have heard before. But you must not be under the illusion that we can do it for you. This book will explain what is happening to you and why. It will teach you how to control the factors which lead to PFR, and how to lose that unwanted weight – but you have to do it!

Let us start by telling how we discovered the PFR Syndrome.

We run a computer-based health and personal growth system, Life Profile Ltd. Basically, what it does is to ask clients where they are now, what sort of state they are in, and where they would like to be, what sort of condition they would like to achieve. We found that the Life Profile computers produced a series of very similar patterns for clients with slimming problems which had common features. Computers are very good at producing such patterns.

In providing individual programmes for slimming and weight loss we noticed two things. One we had anticipated; but the other was a surprise. The first was the problem which everyone who tries to lose weight by dieting alone quickly discovers: that while you can lose weight in this way, keeping it off is very difficult. To overcome this we tended to avoid conventional diets, concentrating instead on guiding people towards a healthy balanced way of eating. To enable them to slim we adjusted their life pattern and activity level. By and large this is a successful strategy; most of our clients achieved their desired weight and physical condition, and found little difficulty in maintaining it.

But at the same time, there were clients who, whatever we recommended, could not lose weight, or could not keep it off. Most were women who, although no more likely than men to suffer from weight problems, are generally more aware of them and find it more difficult to shed fat. We have aimed this book primarily at women, because they are more likely to become victims of PFR for reasons that will be explained later. However, men too can suffer from PFR, and it is likely that the same mechanism is capable of producing other serious effects in men; these are explored in the epilogue.

Every now and then, clients would report sudden weight increases that occurred over a fairly short period of time and for no obvious reason. They accumulated body fat at what was for them an alarming rate.

We knew that this tended to happen to conventional slimmers; the whole see-saw of weight loss followed predictably by weight gain was exposed in *Dieting Makes You Fat* by Geoffrey Cannon and Hetty Einzig. But our system had been specifically designed both to cope with individual variability and to avoid this trap. So what was going wrong?

Two things stood out. Some women proved unable to keep fat off, even if they ate almost nothing at all. And others who appeared to have solved their body weight problem would suddenly put on excess weight. This weight increase happened for no reason that the information at our command could explain, and to complicate matters further, once this mystery fat had gone on, it proved very difficult to shift.

Obviously something was happening which had not been suspected before. We started to isolate the data we had on clients who seemed to be victims, and put them on to a special computer programme to see if we could identify the cause. We called the problem the Persistent Fat Retention Syndrome – because that is exactly what it is.

We read many books and scientific papers in our search for clues. An outline of the problem was sent to the experts who have contributed to the Life Profile data base. It was a little like asking all your friends to give you ten pieces of their favourite jigsaw puzzle, and then trying to put them all together! Nevertheless, a faint pattern did begin to emerge. As in all puzzles once solved, the clues are obvious now. There were the reports of DDT being found in the fat of arctic seals; the mysterious mass deaths of seabirds on migratory flights; a sentence in Geoffrey Cannon and Hetty Einzig's book: 'For a while a series of malaises and infections made me feel as if running were in some way literally jogging poisons in my body to the surface', which had echoes in the experience of some Life Profile clients. And the key was staring us metaphorically in the face.

We have long known about the adverse effects of prescription drugs. Our first book, *Cured to Death*, highlighted the horrifying situation revealed by our research in this field. Despite this, it was not until one of our clients gave us information that related her dramatic accumulation of fat with a particular course of drug treatment that the whole puzzle fell into place.

After careful checking and consultation, we developed a new programme for those Life Profile clients who were victims of the PFR Syndrome. It solved the problem.

This book is the result of this work. We believe that if you are one of the millions of women who struggle continually with unwanted fat, who have found no permanent answer to the diet see-saw, you could be a victim of this syndrome. Here is your answer!

CHAPTER 2

The Calorie Conundrum

It is a startling fact that British society as a whole is eating less than ever before – apart from those times we have experienced famine. Over the past two decades the average calorie consumption per day in Britain has dropped from 2,628 to 2,180, a fall of ten per cent per decade. The textbooks on food requirements have to be periodically revised as the statistics prove that we can live on much less than the experts proclaimed.

Yet at the same time the British people – along with those of other Western nations – are getting fatter and heavier than ever before. In 1980, a woman of average height (5ft 4in) weighed three-quarters of a stone more than she would have done in 1930 or 1943. On average, men too have gained close on a stone. This increase represents the greater quantity of fat with which our bodies are now burdened. In the United States, and probably also in Britain, the average person has ten per cent more fat than twenty years ago!

Although there will be many individual exceptions to this general picture, it represents an undeniable trend towards each of us accumulating fat as time goes by. The traditionally angular, phlegmatic British are turning into a nation of chubbies. Yet the superficial observer would expect exactly the opposite.

Tens of millions of people diet in Britain. Two out of every three women are either dieting or between one diet and the next. And despite the fact that dieting is not an effective answer, more and more men are joining the self-depriving and suffering hordes. On top of this, millions have taken up exercise. Aerobites and dancers gyrate and burn, panting joggers pound the streets, and every town worth its salt substitute has its civic Marathon.

According to the conventional wisdom, all of this effort and activity should be reducing our weight. We are taught that the fewer calories we eat, the less fat we will put on. Obesity experts and the multi-million pound slimming industry agree: the way to get slim is by following a low calorie diet.

Not only is this simplistic nonsense, as most of us know from bitter experience, but, as we shall show later, it is a view that brings with it many dangers for health without any advantages. The truth is that for many of us the fat we carry is only very loosely connected with our calorie intake, whether this is excessive or not. The usual result of this approach is that, even though a reduction in food intake is reflected in short-term weight loss, that weight goes right back on – often in greater quantities – the second will-power flags or something disrupts the diet obsession.

For those who have added exercise to their armoury in the fight against flab the situation is frequently not much better. They may be fitter, but are they less fat? Many people find that, despite burning calories by the score, they keep more fat than they would like. Indeed, they put on weight, because the physical effort to burn off fat becomes so great that they find they are building muscle. For any hope of success, such a slimming routine needs to be very finely tuned and as obsessively followed as the slimmer's diet.

The exerciser's hopes are dashed almost as frequently as those of the dieter. Why is this? Although exercise and activity have much to recommend them as main parts of a conventional slimming strategy, they are limited by the same understanding that governs dieting: input in calories must be less than output in energy. We are back to the simple old calorie equation that conspicuously fails for large numbers of people.

The most serious criticism of the calorie-fat equation is not merely that it is demonstrably inadequate, but that, for any hope of success no matter how limited, it demands total dedication. It requires that slimmers who seriously accept calorie control as their means of salvation become quite literally obsessed.

Slimness should not be such a difficult thing to achieve. Humans are naturally active animals. To have achieved our position of dominance over other species, we must have led naturally healthy lives without becoming excessively fat. There is no doubt that if we are slim we are fitter and healthier; this is our optimum natural state.

Our body has a whole range of complex and subtle mechanisms for maintaining all its systems at their best constant level. Our temperature is the best example; it varies only when something is going wrong. Similarly, our body weight will tend to be maintained at a level which is naturally best for us. There will be seasonal variations, a little fat to carry us through the winter, and changes that fit our changing roles as we grow older. But by and large our capacity for homoeostasis – that is, retaining a constant state – will dictate that we tend to revert to our most efficient weight.

So what is going wrong? The slimmer's obsessive fight to override the body's efforts to put on fat would seem to indicate that what our bodies think best is in direct conflict with our beliefs and wishes. Fighting to assert our desires in preference to our bodies' priorities is bound to be damaging to health.

A wild exaggeration? We think not. The harm is caused by a basic misunderstanding of what happens to our bodies when we try to lose fat, whether by dieting or by combining diet and exercise. In fact, instead of reducing fat, these efforts cause the body to metabolize lean tissues. Why should it behave so apparently illogically? If fat were simply a passive store of excess calories, why should valuable and active tissue from muscles and vital organs be shed in preference to fat?

In failing to ask – or answer – these questions, all those who have offered answers to people who wish to lose weight have been missing a major point. Fat must be far more than an accidental accretion that happens to annoy us, and that we can casually get rid of.

Offering diets which will allow adherents to believe they can eat more yet weigh less by choosing substances which pass through digestive tracts with minimal effect, is a hopeless task. It ignores the physiological needs that are fulfilled by correct nourishment, and assumes that our metabolic processes are easily fooled.

Similarly, those who offer a way of changing or correcting supposed metabolic imbalances with medicines or other substances are clutching at straws. Such a major and widespread trend, in which the metabolic processes of millions of individuals are actually fighting to maintain fat, is unlikely to be amenable to such tinkering.

Nor has medicine been of much help to those who have ended up with problems of severe obesity. Most doctors are locked in the calorie-equals-fat era. In desperation some have even resorted to wiring up the jaws of obesity sufferers. When people agree to be treated in this way, surely something is desperately wrong with our understanding, both of ourselves and of what is happening to us?

The problem of excess weight is not limited to those who want to look good on the beach. It is spreading throughout the age range in our society. By the age of eleven, when traditionally they are as stringy as beanpoles, eight per cent of boys and ten per cent of girls are more than twenty per cent over the normal reference weight for their height. According to *Nutrition Reviews*, the average weight of Americans in relation to their height is continuing to rise. We think it would be difficult to blame this on bad eating habits in the accepted sense.

There are signs that some professionals in the field are beginning to come to terms with some of the puzzles and illogicalities of our increasing weight. In the *International Journal of Obesity*, G. A. Bray noted 'obesity may be a collection of diseases with multiple aetiology'; in other words many things can cause obesity. The cynical interpretation of this remark would be that it is an admission both that the experts have been wrong, and that they admit they do not understand. A more positive view is that it accepts that people are all different, and will be affected by different things in different ways. Unless a solution to unwanted weight addresses itself to this fact, it is likely to fail.

Our increasing problems with fat have many puzzling features. Even the Royal College of Physicians has recently admitted that 'the traditional view that the majority of over-weight subjects are eating more or exercising less than those of a normal weight is now recognized as not being uniformly true'. But until we have a clearer picture of the reality, we are not likely to be able to solve the problem.

While we must not forget the importance of individual differences, it is possible to identify some general features.

For millions, slimming efforts based on conventional under-standing of the body's fat mechanisms fail.

We are eating less, yet weighing more.

Many people find that they can put on large amounts of fat at an alarming rate.

If pressured into losing weight, the body will frequently shed healthy lean tissue rather than apparently inert fat.

Excess fat is neither healthy nor natural, but our bodies insist on creating and maintaining it.

So what are we to conclude?

The answer seems inescapable. Something is causing our bodies to believe that it is in their best interests to put on fat. And whatever forces promote this belief in our metabolic systems, they are already widespread and becoming increasingly common.

The questions we now have to answer are these. Why do our bodies need this extra fat? What is the mechanism that forces them to maintain it? And what can we do about it?

CHAPTER 3

Take a New Look at Fat

This chapter is not intended to persuade you to come to terms with your fat or to accept your body as it is. Slim people do tend to be healthier and more successful, and we should all aim to be at our optimum weight, with no unnecessary fat.

But, as we concluded in the last chapter, our bodies seem to believe quite emphatically that they need fat – much more fat than makes sense to us. And our metabolic systems will go to extreme lengths to make or preserve our fat.

To understand why this is so we need to look at the reasons why our bodies make fat. If you cannot bear to wait for an explanation of the PFR Syndrome, go straight to chapter 6; but if you are serious about permanently losing that weight, just read on – there is no substitute for detailed knowledge of your enemy!

Fat cells are laid down very early in life, mostly before we are born. When our weight increases in adulthood, these cells are pumped up with fat and water; we don't actually grow new cells, but rather those we have are filled. They have an enormous capacity for expansion.

Fat has a wide range of functions in our lives, ranging from effects on the psychology of reproduction to the molecular management of our metabolism. The amount of fat we carry depends on the mixture of its functions that are important to us as individuals at any particular time, balanced against the costs that may be incurred by our bodies in maintaining extra weight.

This is a complex interaction which will vary according to circumstances and at each stage of our lives.

To simplify the picture we can split fat functions into four areas. These are:

1. Sexual attraction
2. Insulation
3. Food storage
4. Neutralization of poisons

While the first three may be familiar to you, it is the fourth function which is at the heart of the problem of persistent fat retention. The discovery that fat has this function is entirely new. It is the crucial explanation for the fat and cellulite problems experienced by so many women. It explains the puzzles of the previous chapter.

But it would be misleading, not to say irresponsible, if we were to encourage you to think that, armed with an understanding of this function, you could solve your weight problem. All of the functions of fat will be important to you to some degree. And the importance of each will have a different emphasis for different people. No single simple answer will work for us all. What we must aim for is our own answer, with the right balance of each of these functions for our needs. With the balance right we can then safely lose fat and be slim and healthy.

1 Fat and sexual attraction

In our culture we tend to overlook the fact that fat plays an important part in making women sexually attractive. The rounded and shapely contours displayed by pin-up models are formed by that subcutaneous layer of fat peculiar to the female; and breasts, the hallmark of femininity, are almost entirely composed of fatty tissues.

It is well known that some African and Arabian societies have taken the sexual implications of fat to the extreme. For them the fatter the bride, the more her worth, and dances and displays have been devised to show off plump behinds or well-covered bellies to best advantage. And whatever the public attitudes of our culture, it remains true that large women seem to have little difficulty in attracting men.

At the other extreme, the slimmers' disease, anorexia nervosa, is a growing phenomenon which reflects deep and widespread problems about self-acceptance, especially among adolescent girls. The changes that take place in the shape of young girls' bodies as they approach maturity act as signals. To males, the feminine accumulation of fatty tissue in the 'right' places says 'I am sexually mature and ready to be approached.' To other females, the message is 'I am no longer a child; I am ready to be treated as an equal.' Such messages may not always be welcome because they indicate irrevocable change, both for the individual girl and for her social relationships. When combined with other physical manifestations, the growth of body hair and the beginning of menstruation, the whole experience can be quite overwhelming. This is especially difficult when it happens against a background of heavy parental inhibition and sexual guilt, or an antagonistic relationship between mother and daughter.

The girl is driven into maturity by forces outside her control. But at some level she is aware of the role of fat; it is the re-shaper of her girlish innocent body, and periods and fertility are only initiated when she achieves a certain height/weight ratio. Without needing to understand these processes, she can perceive that they are associated with fat. The solution to these unwanted changes – self-starvation – can seem fatally obvious.

From these tragically extreme cases it is not a difficult step to see the need to be perpetually slimming as a diluted form of sexual role rejection. Some men, who find the overt sexuality of the mature woman threatening, encourage this behaviour and reinforce the underlying anxiety. And those who fail to make the effort, for whatever reason, are made to carry a burden of guilt for not striving to attain the slim silhouette we are all supposed to desire.

Too many women have lives which are tangled and tied by these twin knots of guilt. One teaches us to reject our femininity and sexuality; the other traps us into self-rejection if we do not conform to an ideal notion of how we should be. And there we stay for decades, one part of the trap reinforcing the other, while success eludes us because our motives are hidden by our upbringing and our culture. We are neither free nor accepted.

Men who put on fat are almost equally rejected. With their feminized bodies, they have difficulty finding partners – which can be very distressing for the twenty-five per cent of young men who are overweight.

The background values of our culture magnify the pain inherent in this situation. If you are overweight, you are ugly, and that is because you eat too much. You may not actually eat a lot, but in terms of your own body you are greedy, and that as we all know is a very near cousin of that sin, gluttony. From there the ethical trap can be extended in almost any direction you may wish. Fat people are not only greedy, they are also obviously lazy – they won't make the effort to balance input with output as conventional wisdom says they should. It is all too easy to surround fat with values that in effect destroy the lives of those who are its victims. From uncertain sexuality we can end up with total self-rejection and destruction.

2 Fat as Heat Insulation

We live in the temperate zone of the world. It goes without saying that our climate is extremely variable and very fickle. Our bodies have adapted by being able to put on fat quickly in times of plenty, and to lose it slowly and cautiously as needed or when the summer returns. Fat is an essential part of our survival repertoire, but today, when life is not so harsh, this ability is not appreciated.

If you are courageous enough to let your weight fluctuate as it will over the course of a year, a logical pattern should emerge. In the winter you will put on fat, then you'll lose it slowly as the days lengthen and the temperatures rise. Try on last year's shorts at Easter and you may be distressed by those bulges above and below; if you resist the panic and carry on as though you didn't care, the chances are that by the hot days of midsummer you'll look as good in them as you did last summer.

In the late autumn, when the winds wake up, the days shorten and temperatures fall, we miss the fat that seemed to melt away in those long, hot summer days. The nagging desire for food intensifies; at times you feel you may blow away if you don't get some food inside you. If you are confident enough to respond to your body's needs, you will accept the hunger, eat and put on weight as the weather turns colder. A little more fat will insulate your internal organs from the stress of the cold so that you can function more effectively, indoors as well as out.

Most of us do follow this natural pattern. Statistics on average calorie consumption – a guide to how much we eat, not to how much fat we put on – show that we eat most in the last three months of the year, and least from April to June.

Those who absolutely reject this natural cycle lose out in two ways. Fighting the body's desire for some winter fat is to do battle with all the inclinations of your metabolism. It is very stressful. Like all stress, it may have a variety of secondary health effects, from raised blood pressure to reduced resistance to infections. You may keep off a few pounds, but you will risk paying a high price in health. And you will lose also in enjoyment, for you will feel the cold. You will be huddled up to the heat while your more realistic friends can enjoy the crisp air, perhaps skiing or doing other winter sports. If you give your body all the wrong messages, it will respond accordingly. It won't keep itself warm, it won't guard against infections as it should and it certainly will not give you the energy you envy in others.

We are designed to cope with cold by putting on fat. A little more insulation tells our system all is well. And this need is not a superficial one that can be switched off by a fashionable diet, pill or exercise routine. White, northern races survived the last Ice Age because of this ability; it is not a lesson our genes will forget easily, nor will they let us forget it.

Indeed, many of us are so highly tuned to this response that a sudden drop in temperature during the day can push us towards the kitchen. Of course, this urge will be heightened for those who are already fighting off the fat, and may help tip them over the edge into a binge. This in its turn will lead them into guilt, which will only make them more susceptible to another unintended binge. It is a problem that can be easily avoided by a more understanding approach.

Those who have studied the variations in body sizes between different races of the world have found that there is a consistent relationship between latitude and body weight. In general, the further away from the equator are our origins, the shorter and stockier we will be. In the hottest regions people tend to grow very long and thin: in some African tribes the men are seven feet tall, with long legs and skinny bodies – probably the roots of many American basketball players.

The long, thin body shape loses heat more efficiently. Further away from the equator the increasing roundedness of the body helps to conserve heat. This is because shorter, more rounded shapes have less surface area to radiate the heat. Although we can't alter the type of body we have, living in chilly conditions will tend to make us plumper than living in warmer climates. As those California girls should know, just living in a warm climate tends to keep you slim, whether you follow an esoteric fruit diet or not. And the same general rule is true for all of us, because the environment will have that effect on our physical make-up.

An easy test to discover how fat acts as an insulator is to feel the different parts of your body in a slightly cool room, say just before you get dressed. Your buttocks will feel relatively cold compared to your upper back, and other areas will show similar differences. Generally, the effect is to insulate the core of your body, where all the vital organs are. As the womb, of course, comes high on the list, covering the bony girdle of the hips is a natural priority for the female body.

Recent research suggests that people with weight problems are not able to use fat for heating as effectively as leaner people. Some scientists believe that they lack the special type of fat, brown adipose tissue or brown fat, that produces heat fastest. This may be because dieters lose brown fat more quickly than fat which fulfils other functions. The body seems to sacrifice cold protection capacity by losing brown fat. This would explain why dieters often feel cold even though they have obvious stores of insulating fat on their bodies, and why their metabolic processes are less likely to respond to sudden cold by burning fat.

3 Fat as a Food Store

Everyone knows that we store excess food as fat. In fact, this is taken so much for granted that many imagine it to be the only function of fat.

The fact that the medical profession has consistently looked at fat in this way for the last century may explain the general ineffectiveness of its approach to obesity and anorexia. Doctors, in concert with the other 'experts', assert that fat develops as a result of the calorie equation being wrong; fat is a passive store of excessive input.

The reason for the persistence of this limited and blinkered view is that it is partially true; the storage of excess food is one function of fat. But that is very different from saying, or behaving as if, calorie storage is the only function of fat.

If you are grossly overweight, it is quite possible that you could lose a lot of your excess by a simple calorie control approach. Because if you persist in eating more than you need it will be stored as fat, and this store can in some cases be used up with little trouble. But you will find that the use of fat stores is subject to the law of diminishing returns. As you lose weight by calorie control, it becomes progressively harder to shed more weight by the same method.

Those who have tried to slim by calorie control alone will have discovered for themselves the very obvious and distressing limits of this view of fat. Even if you live for years on minimal calories, it is still possible to have a disproportionately large amount of fat on your body. So what are the realistic limits of this approach?

A store of fat in excess of that required for female shaping and heat insulation, is considered desirable by the metabolism of women of reproductive years. Once more there is an inescapable survival logic behind this tendency. If, having become attractive and shapely, you then in the nature of things become pregnant, your body wants to ensure that you have enough reserves to get you and the baby through nine months.

While women are sexually active, the body will try to keep a little extra fat on, if only as an insurance policy against damage to a possible baby. This protection will be maintained throughout adulthood. If for any reason this store gets too small, the hormones tend to diminish sexual desire.With further weight loss menstruation will cease, ovulation will become erratic, and the chances of successful conception and pregnancy will be dramatically reduced.

So we have another paradox for the obsessive slimmer who claims attraction of the opposite sex as her motivation. Is she really that easily fooled or is she just fooling herself?

Most women will be in the traumatic hunger zone if they try to reduce their calorie intake below the level at which their bodies can maintain adequate reserves to meet the contingencies of pregnancy. And if you and your body disagree on what is an adequate reserve, you face the misery of a life-long battle with yourself – at least while you are capable of reproducing.

Because reproduction is of primary importance in biological terms, dieting to below this level of fat can be dangerous. Essentially it amounts to this: if your body has to choose between your well-being and the survival of your potential child, the scales will tip in favour of your child.

In practical terms this means that if you insist on losing weight below the level your body feels is right, you will not lose fat: you will lose lean tissue. This will be in the form of muscle, and also tissue from vital organs: liver, kidneys and heart. Your body will start to destroy you to protect your possible baby's chances. The pictures of unfortunate famine victims illustrate this in action; women who are obviously starving still have enough fat to maintain their breasts and feed their babies – these are the last systems to be shut down by starvation.

Over the decades many millions of women have subjected themselves to this destructive process, usually without realizing it. What they have observed is that after losing weight in this way, they tend to put fat on more rapidly than before. They are on the dieter's see-saw; dieting actually makes them fat.

With each rise in body weight, the proportion of fat carried increases. When their weight is shed, they tend to lose a greater proportion of lean tissue and a classic vicious circle is set up. People who have been the victims of this are more likely to end up as sufferers of the PFR Syndrome because the lost liver tissue is one route into the syndrome. We will explain how and why later.

Before considering the final function of fat, it may be useful to summarize the points we have covered so far. We shall be breaking new ground, so it is a good idea to make sure that the old is in perspective before doing this.

Fat, hated or not, is essential to body functions, particularly for women. It forms the body shape we recognize as typically feminine. It provides heat insulation, keeping our vital organs warm and giving protection for babies. It also provides the body weight necessary for reproduction; women of reproductive age will be pushed to carry spare fuel in the form of fat to ensure their babies have the best chance of survival. Beyond this critical fat level, some surplus food may get put into store in the form of fat.

The reasons we have evolved to use fat in these ways are fairly straightforward. Fat is relatively inactive in metabolic terms; as you know, it tends just to be there, so it does not require much energy for maintenance. The metabolic rate of people with high proportions of fat in their bodies is much lower than that of people with less fat and more muscle. This means that women, with higher fat proportions than men, need less food to keep them alive, and plumper women actually need less than their leaner sisters. And this is another factor which gives them, and their children, an extra edge for survival.

So the survival needs of our species drive us in a circle. Fat makes women distinctively female, and signals their arrival at maturity. At some level men understand that fat means better chances for the survival of their children, and go along with the pattern reinforced by our evolutionary experience. So the daughters of women who use their fat effectively, for sexual attraction and survival, will tend to perpetuate the process. They carry the genes for a 'thrifty' metabolism – one that will function effectively on little food – and they pass them on to their offspring. This is the essence of the survival of the fittest.

Our bodies are still very efficient at adapting to the conditions in which we live; the capacity to change in ways which will maximize our chances of survival is still there. Those adaptations we have been discussing, which made the most of our ancestors' chances over millions of years evolution, still have a few tricks in reserve. While we as town-dwelling, well-clothed, heated, car-using and cared-for individuals for whom food is always available may not appreciate the effects of these survival tricks, we will not be able to control them unless we understand them.

At this point, before the emergence of the PFR Syndrome, it would have been possible to draw up a comprehensive strategy for almost anyone to lose as much weight as they wanted. Indeed, this is what we used to do for Life Profile clients, devising programmes that would shed surplus food stores, then persuade the body it did not need pregnancy reserves or so much insulation.

It was the realization that fat had a fourth function that

caused us to re-write all our programmes. We believe that all serious slimmers need to change their view of fat and its relationship to them just as drastically if they are to control their fat.

4 Fat As A Toxin Store

We know what we mean by fat, but it is important to understand what we mean by a toxin. According to the Concise Oxford Dictionary a toxin is 'a poison especially of animal or vegetable origin'. As when trying to describe other new concepts, the existing definitions reveal their limitations; the PFR Syndrome is no exception. We have to extend the notion of a toxin to mean any substance which the body treats as a poison. It is the way in which the body treats toxins that holds the key to the problem of persistent fat retention.

As we have seen, the conventional view of fat is that it is essentially passive. It sits on the body, shaping by its position, insulating and storing food energy. What we are proposing is that fat also has an active role in the body: that of a storage medium for substances the body regards as toxic. When the body encounters substances which are too toxic to be dealt with in the normal way by the metabolism, they are put into storage. Different types of toxin go into tissues which are best suited to their storage. We know that lead is stored in bones, but the most common poisons we encounter today go into fat. Remember the clue of DDT in the fat of arctic seals?

We would go further. The problem of the PFR Syndrome is that the body will manufacture fat, in large quantities if necessary, and against all efforts to stop it, so that it can store toxins. The case histories in the next chapter illustrate this process quite clearly.

To see how this happens we need to understand a little of how the body makes fat and how it uses it up. The using-up process is disrupted in large numbers of people, locking fat on to their bodies.

When we digest food, it is broken down and reorganized at the molecular level, rearranged into forms that we can use. Our digestive processes are complicated, but this has the advantage of allowing us to survive on almost anything; our bodies rearrange the food molecules into the molecules they want. We can even swap molecules around within our bodies, reusing them in different ways to meet different needs.

Carbohydrates, those foods many slimmers traditionally but erroneously avoid, are broken down into sugars, fibre and other constituents. The sugars and valuable trace components are absorbed, while the complex carbohydrates which we call 'fibre' continue to move through the gut. Proteins, larger and even more complex molecules, are split into smaller molecules called polypeptides, and later into their constituent amino acids – the basic building blocks of life. Fats are broken down into fatty acids and glycerin; fatty acids may be used in various metabolic processes, while glycerin is changed by the liver's enzyme systems into glucose. This can be stored in the liver in the form of glycogen or released into the bloodstream for instant energy.

The liver is the real 'back room' of our body. It does not usually get much publicity or attention, but it should; it performs over twenty major functions, all essential for our wellbeing. The best way to think of the liver is as a vast marshalling yard, with trains constantly coming in and being reformed to take wagons to different destinations. Some traffic will go off and come in by other means: road or water. The whole system is integrated by communications at many levels – signals, sensors and a computer.

All our digested food moves around the body in our blood. From the digestive organs it is carried directly into the liver by the hepatic portal vein, the main input to the marshalling yard where the sorting begins. Now, in addition to all our nutrients, the blood will also be carrying substances we don't want. The liver metabolizes, or breaks down for disposal, such substances; they may range from cancer cells, viruses, the natural products of cellular breakdown, hormones, fat being recycled for energy, to drugs and other foreign substances.

The most usual exit route for unwanted substances is through our kidneys. But these substances have to be made soluble in water before they can be shipped out in this way. For those that cannot be dissolved in water, the next choice is to dissolve them in fat. They are carried in the bile, which is secreted by the liver, into the bile duct and into the digestive tract once more. If they take the hint, these substances are eliminated in solid waste. Unfortunately, this system is not very efficient. To save effort, the endlessly busy liver recycles bile, only losing small amounts as waste, and inevitably some of the garbage gets recycled as well; this is the untidy end of the marshalling yard. There is some advantage in this disorder; the levels of some substances can be kept more or less constant by recirculating; other substances can be recycled, thus saving effort for other systems. The danger is that substances that are totally undesirable are not totally eliminated, and they can build up in the system.

When the liver can't cope, fat-soluble substances go into store to be dealt with later. The store is body fat. The substances which overload the liver will vary from individual to individual. They may range from known poisons, through drugs, to food additives. The molecules concerned will tend to have one thing in common; they are most likely to be the ubiquitous man-made organic molecules that are increasingly common in the twentieth-century environment.

For those whose systems become overloaded, or whose capacity is reduced, an increasing number of substances are likely to be shunted into fat. Whether the liver will be able to cope at a later time is then the crucial question. In the mean-time, the result is the deposit of toxic adipose tissue – or contaminated fat.

Perhaps we should not be surprised that substances the liver can't cope with end up in deposits of fat. The low turnover of tissue reflected in its slow metabolic rate means that any poisons stored in fat can be left undisturbed where they will do least harm. In most parts of the body there is a constant cycle of breakdown and renewal; for example, it is estimated that we replace all the bones of our skeleton every seven years. In fat there is less of this activity. It is accumulated, and there it stays until it is called off for energy. Its insulating and shaping properties are entirely passive, it could be replaced by a wrap of foam or a pad of silicon.

There are other characteristics which make fat an ideal toxin store. As many of us know, it can be put on very quickly, frighteningly fast at times. And it can be put on in large amounts. Because it has a low metabolic rate it does not require much in the way of ancillary servicing; no ligaments, bones, very few nerves, hardly any major blood vessels. The fat cells are there ready to be filled up as required.

Of course, this will not be everyone's experience. The easy deposition of persistent fat will come as news to some. They are the lucky ones. People do vary enormously in many ways, both obviously and very subtly. For some, toxins will be much more readily neutralized by their metabolic processes. The old saying dear to grandmother that one man's meat is another man's poison was correct – one woman's harmless substances may be another's three-stone-weight gain. The 'lucky' ones, confronted with the same substances, will not produce the same stores of fat because they don't need them.

But there are others who are simply not as efficient at dealing with toxins. This may be because of the way they live, or through liver damage, or simply because they started out with a relatively small liver in relation to their body weight. For these individuals, persistent fat retention can take another step; the toxins with which they cannot cope will actually damage their livers, thus further reducing their capacity to cope.

For those who have been on the diet see-saw the loss of liver tissue may be crucial. Their decreased metabolic capacity will make it even more likely that the body will put on fat. And if these people persist in dieting, their livers will become even more inefficient because their limited stores of a crucial de-toxifying substance (glutathione – its role is described in detail in chapter 7) are used up in the effort to maintain the function of the rest of the body.

As the capacity to cope decreases, the metabolism comes to regard more substances as toxic. This is what happens with increasing age; metabolic shocks from which we could bounce up in the vitality of youth can put us to bed for a few days. Under some circumstances, if metabolic capacity continues to decrease, there is a point of no return; the unfortunate alcoholic who dies of cirrhosis of the liver is the most familiar example.

We are not suggesting that persistent fat is a sign of imminent fatality. What we are saying is this; you may be subjecting your systems to a range of subtle influences which have the combined effect of creating a toxic reaction. The protective response of the body to this toxic reaction is to lay down fat to store the toxin. Until you put on the fat, and find you can't shift it, you may not notice anything at all – because this coping mechanism allows you to stay healthy in spite of exposure to high levels of toxic substances.

The changes that make you susceptible to PFR often make little subjective impression. The exception may be when there is an obvious response to marked changes in environmental conditions. The subtle and varying initiators of the condition are factors which made answering the question of why so many slim women suddenly put on weight difficult to answer.

If we accept that fat has a lot to do with our ability to survive, and that this ability has been extended recently to include acting as an active storage medium for harmful toxins, then the process is easier to understand. These women's bodies were acting in the best way they could to protect them from a serious hazard.

As with all fat functions, our bodies tend to overdo it, to err on the side of safety. The problem of being slim is to persuade our bodies that enough is enough, and perhaps a little less than enough would be quite adequate. For the first three functions of fat persuasion is the only successful tactic; for the fourth, once we have become victims of the PFR Syndrome, the only answer is detoxification. Our strategy explains how to do this.

Before going on to case histories which illustrate the PFR Syndrome, it may be time to consider just how widespread it is. We cannot be sure of figures, of course; your individual experience is the best indicator of your position. But we are left wondering if we may not have stumbled across the answer to that large puzzle: could it be that the reason why as a nation we are eating less and less, yet weighing more and more, is that to some degree we are all victims of this syndrome? That our bodies are being called upon to cope with ever more toxins, and increased weight in the form of fat is the only answer to this chemical onslaught?

CHAPTER 4

The PFR Syndrome

The PFR Syndrome is the effect of toxins in body fat. The human body is capable of dissolving a great range of potentially poisonous substances in fat, and of producing fat to store these substances. Toxins which can induce this reaction are very widespread in our environment; we absorb them from our food and from many other sources.

The fat becomes poisoned in the process, and because of this it is very difficult to shed. PFR victims are people who carry excess weight that they find they cannot lose. Their bodies retain stores of persistent fat.

The clearest sign of the PFR Syndrome is a sudden increase in fatty tissue. In this context sudden may mean a few weeks or a period of months. The latter is more likely if you have been consistently trying to lose weight while your body has been trying to put it on.

If you have recently put on weight and now find it will not shift, even though you may have put it on and taken it off quite easily in the past, it is almost certainly a case of PFR.

In addition to obvious fat, cellulite and that less dense, 'watery' flab – typically hanging from the upper arms and thighs – may also be used by the body to store toxic residues. PFR Syndrome victims have bodies which will create deposits of toxic adipose tissue in a variety of sites. All forms of such tissue will be amenable to the same treatment.

Have you, before or during a period of weight gain, been

exposed to anything in your environment which your body may regard as toxic? It may be that in the absence of any direct and sudden exposure, your system is responding adversely to a low level of build-up over a long time. This is particularly likely if you've been dieting or unwell.

Some drugs are known to cause weight gain. If you have recently taken a course of medication for a particular problem, say depression, and found yourself putting on unexplained weight, that is characteristic of the PFR Syndrome. Similarly, taking oral contraceptives will make you more susceptible to it. A wide range of other substances have been noted as causal factors, but because of individual variability it is impossible to give a comprehensive check list. Your own experience after use or exposure is the best guide to their effects on you.

One effect that may be noticeable after exposure to a toxin is an unusual desire for sweet or fatty foods. Your body may be demanding those substances that can be directly routed into fat stores, and it can be an indication that your liver has opted to dump something it does not like into fat.

Other signs of toxic exposure that may lead to persistent fat retention are such things as: an outbreak of spots; brittle nails; an unseasonal shedding of hair. These can mean that the body is struggling to get rid of substances it does not like. Spots may be the immune system working to shed matter through the skin, while nail and hair growth require proteins related to those urgently needed by the liver for detoxification.

The role of the liver is crucial in the PFR Syndrome. Small people will tend to be more at risk, simply because they have smaller livers. A rough guide to the efficiency of your liver is the effect alcohol has on you. Some victims have reported getting drunk on one or two small drinks, and a nasty hangover from one more. Obviously, their livers were not coping too well. Other signs are that physical effort tends to produce a feeling of cold or hangover some time later.

Similarly, people who have some other condition, such as allergies, which indicates some malfunction with either the immune system or liver metabolism, will be more at risk. This group includes those who suffer from arthritis and other auto-immune diseases as well as hay fever, asthma and food allergy. The Plan we suggest in chapter 9 will help, both by reducing susceptibility to such conditions, and reducing the risk of PFR.

Lastly we must consider those people who have been fat for years, and may have given up hope of getting that weight off. For many women this is associated with having children. From the attractive person they were before pregnancy, too often they develop that matronly shape that people are polite about – but which they would rather not have. It is usually assumed that the change in routine associated with being a mother is the cause of this change – but is it? If they have been depriving themselves of food in a long-term effort to contain the weight gain, they will be more at risk because they will have been interfering with their detoxifying systems.

During pregnancy, the liver and kidneys, as well as everything else, work for two. This in itself is a strain, but one we are designed to manage. If you add to it environmental toxins, however, you could be on the edge of a PFR problem. The final factor which may tip pregnant women over the edge is the range of drugs they may be given during the actual birth. Anaesthetics are particularly troublesome for our metabolism, and in an already overloaded state they could be the last straw. For some women, each successive pregnancy adds to the problem. Of course, this might apply to other operations – one of our clients has been tubby ever since a hysterectomy.

It may be that you are one of those people who can lose most of their fat by either diet or exercise, but finds that whatever you do, a particular lump will not shift. A common PFR pattern in these cases is that people become slim all over – except for a layer of fat on their bellies. It can occur in other parts of the body; it depends on the distribution of your most reactive fat cells.

Similarly, you may find that you can lose fat, but only up to a certain point. You need to decide what sort of fat your body is hanging on to, and why. Could it be toxic adipose tissue? Only you can decide. Check where your body prefers to lose it from: if you are losing sexual shaping, from breasts and hips, while keeping fat elsewhere, this is probably PFR.

If your attempts at slimming or physical activity produce headaches or hangovers, beware. This means that the toxins you have stored in fat are coming back to haunt you. You are a PFR victim, and should follow the Plan. Apart from joint aches and pains, and muscular stiffness from unaccustomed effort, physical activity should not produce effects of this sort. Check that nothing peculiar is wrong if you are worried, but in most cases the answer will be obvious.

Finally, illogical fat loss may be your best overall guide. The diagram overleaf indicates how your body should shed fat. Only you can decide how much fat you have, or need, for each function. If your body does not lose weight in the way indicated, it is because it is expressing some desire to retain fat to protect itself. You then have to remove the need for that protection. The PFR Escape Plan will tell you how to do this.

You should not try to lose fat in other than the order indicated. Although you might lose weight, you would create an unnatural body shape, and persistence with misdirected efforts could put your health at risk.

1 To slim successfully you must first remove toxic adipose tissue. If you do not, it will persist even when you have lost all other fat and it will hinder your efforts to lose weight however you go about it. Once you have got rid of it, you will be able to slim to whatever degree you choose. If you do not deal with it, your body will distort its shape and proportions – not at all a desirable end. Toxic adipose tissue just has to go.

2 Energy storage is the fat function where what and how much you eat, the crude calorie idea, has some relevance. But since the effects of the same type and amount of food, identical numbers of calories, have widely different effects on different individuals, this relevance is limited. Calorie counting and diets based on low calorie intake can damage your health.

Eating beyond need often has an emotional basis and this should be tackled honestly if it is your problem. Thereafter, the answer is to establish eating patterns which fulfil the requirements of body and spirit without producing privation or a need for supplements. This type of conscious eating does not involve hardship. The quantity you eat will then have some direct bearing on the amount of fat you carry as stored energy, as will your activity and metabolic rate.

3 Insulating fat is difficult to deal with for many women for two reasons. First, it is cyclical, responding to annual temperature changes. Second, in women of childbearing age the body will consider it desirable to have some insulating fat to see them and any baby through to birth. Fortunately, the answer to insulating fat is simple: physical activity. By increasing your metabolic rate and capacity you decrease the need for insulation. Additionally, you will alter your hormone profile and so lower your body's precautionary demand; at a certain level of activity, menstruation normally ceases.

Most people are quite happy with some insulating fat. Even perpetually active athletes, such as tennis stars, have a healthy layer.

4 Sexual shaping. There are two ways of reducing the amount of fat used for sexual shaping. One is healthy and safe; the other is not.

Shaping fat can be reduced by extreme activity combined with a rigorously strict lifestyle. Thus we reduce the generation of fat by matching input to output in energy terms, and by altering the body's hormone profile to the degree that it is convinced that such fat is of minimal importance. When activity decreases and the lifestyle is relaxed, the body will put on this fat once more. Because of the activity-centred lifestyle, this way of losing fat is usually without risk; such individuals are extremely fit. It is rare, however; even top-class distance runners like Mary Decker Slaney and Zola Budd have some minimal feminine shaping from their fat.

Sexual shaping can also be reduced by starvation, by metabolic changes, by psychological suffering or by a combination of these factors as in anorexia nervosa. Losing weight in any of these ways is not healthy; people who do so are clinically ill.

5 Extreme efforts to lose fat eventually lead to damage to those parts of the body which require fatty tissue for their function, for example the nervous system and brain. Such misguided efforts can prove fatal.

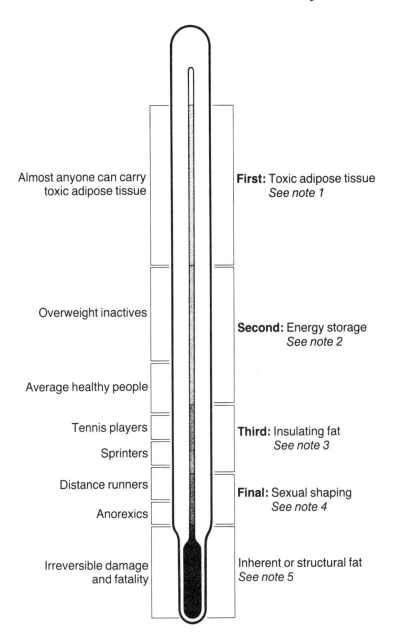

Almost anyone can carry toxic adipose tissue

Overweight inactives

Average healthy people

Tennis players

Sprinters

Distance runners

Anorexics

Irreversible damage and fatality

First: Toxic adipose tissue
See note 1

Second: Energy storage
See note 2

Third: Insulating fat
See note 3

Final: Sexual shaping
See note 4

Inherent or structural fat
See note 5

CHAPTER 5

Case Histories

On her wedding day Amanda Phillips was as slim and pretty as any young woman could wish to be. Small and delicately built, her weight had remained stable at seven stone for almost ten years – ever since her early teens.

Unlike many less fortunate women, she had not had to struggle to achieve this happy state. Staying slim had never been a problem for her; she had no trouble with her appetite, no nagging hunger. And she had always enjoyed energetic sports. She was the sort of person we think of enviably as naturally slim and active.

After Amanda had been married for less than a year she became unaccountably depressed. Looking back now on those black months she still cannot understand what set it all off. We can speculate; the change in lifestyle associated with marriage, an accumulation of small stresses, or perhaps a bad reaction to something in her environment.

Like so many experiencing a sudden and apparently in-explicable change, Amanda consulted her doctor. He could not pin down her problem, but accepted her weepy and miserable symptoms at face value. He took the only action which seemed open to him and prescribed a course of anti-depressant drugs. Amanda took them gratefully.

Her deep depression did not lift immediately, but the doctor explained that the pills often had a delayed effect, and she persisted with the treatment. Gradually her mood changed for the better. In relief at the prospect of returning to her normal happy self, Amanda overlooked the other changes which were happening to her.

All the time, she now felt ravenously hungry and found herself desiring the sort of foods that had never appealed to her before. Suddenly cakes, biscuits and sweets seemed irresistible.

The doctor was reassuring; he explained that an increased appetite was generally considered a healthy sign, probably the consequence of her improved mood. Just as she had lost interest in food during her depression, lifting the depression was almost bound to have the opposite effect. He agreed that she might put on weight, but suggested that this was a small price for the improvement and she would soon lose it again once her depression was completely cured.

Amanda's delicate, girlish figure soon showed the effects, but she and her husband disguised any anxiety by buying new clothes to celebrate her improvement. However, the problem grew too great to ignore; in a few months Amanda had put on three stone.

The excess weight, so quickly gained, proved impossible to lose. Try as she might, Amanda could not rid herself of the fat belly that she had acquired. At first people smiled, assuming she was pregnant. But as the months passed, and she still had that 'six-months-gone' look, it became obvious that this was not the case. The change, and the embarrassment it caused, destroyed her social life.

With the information you already have, what had happened to Amanda may appear obvious. But at the end of the 1970s when this was happening to her, the fourth function of fat, the problem of toxic adipose tissue producing the PFR Syndrome, was simply not suspected. Many pieces of the puzzle were on the table, but nobody had put them together.

Being the sort of person she is, Amanda did not accept her situation. Her first attempts to shift the fat were through dieting. Over a two-year period she tried every diet she could find, and her food intake declined to less than a thousand calories a day. Yet the fat persisted.

She also tried to return to her previous activity level. But this proved impossible, she was simply unable to summon the energy to make it work. The least exertion made her feel desperately tired. She could still swim, but inhibitions about the figure she cut in her costume made the public pool more than she could face. Finally even walking made her feel tired.

Her determination survived, however. Amanda tried exercising in the privacy of her home. She bought aerobics books and tapes, and faithfully followed the exercises, keeping the promise they held firmly in mind. She jogged and twisted to the music of the beginners' routine until sweat ran into her eyes. Gritting her teeth, she fought the desire to drop on to the sofa.

The next day Amanda stayed in bed. She had not felt so ill in her life before. Her head hammered relentlessly, she was weak and felt sick, and her lack of coordination made standing up difficult. It was as though the previous day's exercise had given her an almighty hangover. A week later, when she had recovered, she tried again with the same result. Another week later Amanda tried a little jogging – only to find it gave her a severe headache.

The effort hangover is a common PFR Syndrome symptom. Amanda's experience is a more dramatic form of Hetty Einzig's feeling that she had been jogging poisons into her system when she took up running, described in *Dieting Makes You Fat*. And although it may seem to rule out activity because of its nasty effects, as we shall see later, this reaction among victims can be used as a part of the Plan to beat the syndrome.

It was around this time that Amanda contacted Life Profile and stimulated our search for the answer to her problem. When she wrote Amanda expressed a strong suspicion about the cause of her weight problem; she blamed the course of anti-depressant drugs her doctor had given her. She also reported that she had consulted a variety of specialists; they dismissed her suggestion. While it was conceded that perhaps anti-depressants might cause some temporary weight gain, their opinion was that this weight would come off again. One suggested that Amanda stay in hospital for a week on a monitored diet; he obviously did not believe that she was eating as little as she claimed.

Amanda had tried all the conventional means of losing her excess weight, yet it would not shift. Clearly some mechanism was binding that unwanted fat to her body in a way which had not previously been suspected. The problem we were confronted with was to find out how this mechanism might work; if we could discover what was going on, the hope was that it could be reversed.

We started by taking her suspicion seriously and consulting the medical information on anti-depressant drugs. The literature on these drugs does note weight gain as a common side-effect. It is an effect which has been investigated by psychiatrists, some of whom perceptively observed that this supposedly minor reaction was capable of making its victims even more depressed than they were before they started the drug therapy. For those who already felt unhappy because they were overweight and unattractive, this sort of side-effect could be enough to tip them towards desperation. It is far from a minor or trivial reaction to drug treatment in such cases.

We could not find any explanation for Amanda's reaction in the medical literature, or for the fact that the fat she had put on was so persistent. Meanwhile, the search of Life Profile records produced some other cases, which although not as extreme, had some things in common with Amanda's experience.

The next part of the puzzle was provided by Beth Jackson. Unlike Amanda, Beth had been fighting a tendency to put on weight ever since her teens. She knew that if she wasn't active, if she didn't watch what she ate, she would put on weight. Once this happened she would deliberately change her habits, perhaps starve herself a bit so that the unwanted weight disappeared again. As she got into her mid-twenties, Beth found that if she put on weight, she had to diet conscientiously and be very active to get it off. She also found that it seemed to go on again with increased ease.

Although it was annoying to have to devote more time and effort to controlling her weight, Beth accepted this as part of the life of a career girl. Over nearly a decade she was able to keep on top of it without too much difficulty, providing nothing caught her off balance. But without realizing it, Beth was on the diet see-saw. Each time she shed weight, she was losing a little more lean tissue, and each time she put on weight she had a higher proportion of fat.

What finally threw Beth was lifting a box of paper in the office. Trouble with a disc in her spine put her on her back in bed for three weeks. During this period she was taking tablets for the pain in her recovering back, and, perhaps out of frustration, she was drinking a lot more than usual. Under these conditions she put on weight very quickly.

When she recovered, Beth went back to her old diet and activity routine. It had always worked for her before, after a long and heavy Christmas, or when she had eaten and drunk to compensate for the breakup of a love affair. This time her routine failed her. For all her efforts, Beth was unable to shift more than a very small amount of the weight she had put on during the months of recuperation from her back trouble.

For a long time, Beth assumed that the reason for her problem had simply been her reduced level of activity. But this explanation didn't make a lot of sense. Why was it, she wondered, that the weight stayed on in spite of a sensible diet and her regular exercise regime? This had never happened to her before, and now at thirty-three, although she knew she was not experiencing any major metabolic change, she wondered if it might be just her age. But a nagging doubt remained. It just didn't feel right.

We looked in detail at Beth's activity and diet habits, and naturally we followed up the drugs she had been taking during the episode with her back. These were non-steriodal anti-inflammatories, of which there are many forms. Their main use is the reduction of chronic pain. There was no general acknow-ledgement that they caused weight gain, although weight gain is common among those who take this type of drug on a regular basis, and it is noted as a side-effect for some members of the group.

It is usually assumed that any weight gain is associated with inactivity caused by the painful conditions for which such drugs are prescribed. Arthritis is the most common reason for such long-term use, and by and large this seemed to be a reasonable explanation for most weight gain associated with these drugs. We were left wondering whether there might not be a little over-simplification in this theory much like the assumption that those who grew fat on anti-depressants did so because their improved mood led them to eat more. While we could under-stand people putting on weight when their arthritis interfered with their mobility, what of those whose problems were with their hands? Why should they tend to grow fat too?

It was Beth's drinking which became the focus of our investi-gation. Not that she drank a lot; most of the time hardly at all, but like most of us she would, every now and then, indulge. She had done so at the time she was taking drugs for her back problem. This caused us to think about what might have been happening in her liver at this time. It was a significant step towards discovering the PFR mechanism.

Christopher Denham's weight problem coincided with the onset of asthma. He had been a small, rather delicate child, susceptible to allergic problems, though these had been com-paratively minor. The onset of asthma during early adulthood came as a frightening new development when he and his family moved into the country. He believes the onset was prompted by the accidental drift of pesticide from aerial spraying into his garden.

Chris had discovered that when his asthma was mild, as it was when he lived in Spain for three months, he had little trouble with his weight. But in periods when he was having more frequent or severe attacks, he would put on weight at an alarming rate. Then, when his asthma was controlled with sodium chromoglycate, the problem of weight gain persisted.

We know that many allergic problems, such as hay fever, are basically caused by pollution. Not necessarily the pollution that we acknowledge – the dirt, litter, smoke and fumes that are so offensive – but also the myriad of 'safe' chemical products which are so common in our modern world. Most of these artificial substances are those organic molecules that the liver marshals into fat. Was Chris's case giving us a direct clue? If pollution (with the sudden overload of pesticide, a type of chemical absolutely suitable for both allergic reaction and fat deposition) caused his asthma, might it not also be linked to his weight cycles?

We were almost convinced.

Donna had struggled with weight and fitness throughout her teens and early twenties. Her Life Profile course had enabled her to achieve stable weight and an active life, and she and her husband were happily working to set themselves up before starting a family.

Then suddenly she put on weight very rapidly. Like some other apparent stable clients, she had lost balance. We were trying to solve these clients' problems on an individual basis, assuming that there was no common thread, when we began to consider the possibility of the PFR Syndrome.

The key to Donna's rapid weight gain was similar to that we subsequently recognized in other cases: exposure to a different environment with a particular range of new chemical hazards. Donna started work in an electrical accessory factory. Industry generally has become reliant on the use of new synthetic organic materials; the electrical industry uses them to coat wires for insulation, to make boards for printed circuits and for a wide range of other processes. During manufacture, quantities of these materials are released into the atmosphere, to be breathed in or absorbed through the skin.

The common experience in our cases had now emerged. They had all been exposed to one or more toxic substances. Just how this precipitated their PFR Syndrome is the subject of the next chapter.

CHAPTER 6

PFR – The Cause

PFR is caused by exposure to toxic substances which the victim's metabolism copes with by dumping into toxic adipose tissue. To justify this conclusion we have to go back to our earlier definition of a toxic substance as any substance which the body treats as a poison.

In the cases described in the last chapter, the victims had been exposed to toxic substances in quantities greater than their metabolic processes could deal with. Their bodies had reacted by dumping the excess into fat, laying down more as required to store these toxins safely. This fat was then protected and maintained by the body so that it persisted despite all their efforts to shift it. To use it would mean flooding the system with toxins once more.

This statement may surprise some readers. What toxic substance had Amanda been exposed to? She had become depressed, was prescribed drug therapy and had put on weight. Where do toxins figure in this case?

Most people do not think of medicines as poisons. We are accustomed to concentrating only on their beneficial effects. We forget that there is no such thing as a safe drug; it is easy to overlook the fact that drugs are almost always chemicals which are foreign to the human body, and are at the least regarded as suspicious substances by our metabolic processes. Pharmacologists, who study drugs, and toxicologists, who study poisons, agree that drugs are poisons administered in small doses. All drugs are capable of causing damage to the human body. The quantity which the body will accept without protest or signs of poisoning will vary, from one substance to another and from one individual to another.

So a normal therapeutic dose of any medicine may prove entirely beneficial to one person – yet life-threatening to another. Fortunately, the latter response is rare. The testing carried out is intended to reduce the frequency of such events. Nevertheless, even the safest drugs kill people and cause a wide variety of unwanted adverse reactions or side-effects. Amanda was a victim of one of these adverse reactions.

Amanda's anti-depressant drugs did not make her ill because, although her systems were clearly not coping well enough for the drug to be harmlessly eliminated, a second line of defence had come into operation. Her body had manufactured stores of fat where the potentially damaging substance, or more likely, derivatives from its partial metabolization, had been dumped. This would protect the other organs of her body, such as her heart, from exposure to an overdose.

Her PFR resulted from the fact that any attempt to use that fat would put the toxic drug derivatives back into circulation. Her body would then react in exactly the same way it did the first time it was exposed to these substances – and put them straight back into fat. It seemed that whatever she did, that fat had become firmly attached to her body.

The hangovers she experienced with exercise were just that – hangovers caused by the toxins in her circulation affecting other organs of her body. She recovered when most of the toxin was back in fat stores once more.

Beth's problem is less clear-cut. Inactivity, anti-inflammatory drugs and alcohol all contributed. On the face of it, inactivity caused by her back problem seems the obvious culprit. But that does not explain why the weight would not come off again. Her PFR was the result of a pattern of events which at a particular point in her life, under particular circumstances, produced this effect. Her see-saw dieting over the years had probably reduced the capacity of her liver through lean tissue loss. Thereafter, combining drugs and alcohol would have tended to overload her detoxification system. If she had been her normal active self her system might have coped, but being flat on her back could have been the last straw – her body opted to store its overload in fat.

While it is impossible to be absolutely sure, this interpretation seems to fit all the facts. Though why Beth's body should choose to continue with this option once she became active again is not clear. Whatever the precise route to the problem, there can be no doubt that Beth became a sufferer of the PFR Syndrome.

Beth's case reveals another source of the PFR problem: if anything lowers our capacity, or subjects it to a temporary overload, our metabolism can switch to a different coping system. Clearly, if a variety of factors are priming it and pushing it towards switching, the nature of the last straw involved becomes less critical and consequently more difficult to identify. We will look at the wider sources of potential priming factors for the PFR Syndrome later.

Beth's metabolic switch shows the danger of overload due to a range of potential toxins, interacting with lifestyle factors. It is almost as if the metabolism learns a new trick and then finds it preferable to the old – a very human reaction after all! But this is only conjecture; few processes in the body can be explained with reference to a single mechanism working in one way, and in apparent isolation. Usually a combination of things are at work at many levels to produce the effects we become aware of. This flexibility is a part of the wonder of our being.

Similarly, the reason for unusual sensitivity to unwanted drug effects is often unknown. It is generally assumed that it has to do with variations in the efficiency and balance of enzyme systems which are involved in detoxification. This brings us back to the liver, where these enzymes are produced and do their work, rearranging and disposing of the substances involved. If the systems in a person's body are unable to deal with drugs or other substances at the rate at which they arrive at the liver, then the quantities build up. Eventually they will reach toxic levels.

Christopher's susceptibility to allergic problems was established before he was exposed to the particular episode that apparently precipitated his asthma. It happened to be exposure to large amounts of a pesticide in the air, but it could equally well have been any one of a wide range of substances now circulating in our environment. The substances which load a person to the point where allergies such as eczema, hay fever and asthma are triggered are numerous and widespread. This is why these conditions are increasingly common. It remains true that pesticides, a billion gallons of which are now sprayed on to our land and food each year, are frequently associated with this sort of reaction. In their London offices, Friends of the Earth have thick dossiers of case histories of such individuals.

The essence of an allergic reaction is that the body treats a substance which it may have previously regarded as safe, as dangerous or poisonous. This change of reaction may occur at many levels, involving both the immune and detoxification systems. In hay fever sufferers, the mast cells – the gatekeepers of the immune system – which line membranes exposed to the air, confuse harmless pollen grains with dangerous organisms; while similar mast cells in the gut of food allergy sufferers falsely identify food components as poisonous.

The general feature of allergic conditions is that common substances which are harmless to the majority of people are treated as poisonous by the sufferer's system. The immune and detoxification systems of the body can become stretched in dealing both with these pseudo-poisons and with the treatments that may be taken to counter their effects.

Allergy itself can cause weight gain in some sufferers. The clinical ecologist Richard Mackarness has commented that a cereal-free diet developed for weight loss, which worked despite the fact that it was not low in calories, produced its effects through the elimination from the diet of substances which provoked allergy.

Another clue to the PFR mechanism was provided in Dr Mackarness's book *Not All in the Mind*. In it he describes how Dr Pennington was given the task of developing a weight reducing plan for executives of the Du Pont chemical company. He 'came to the conclusion that obesity in some people is caused by an inability to use carbohydrates for anything except making surplus fat. He . . . postulated a short cut into the fat stores with subsequent difficulty in getting the fat out again for conversion into energy.'

For those whose route into the PFR Syndrome is through an allergic reaction, it makes no difference whether we would recognize the substance they are allergic to as a toxin or not. What is important is that their body deems the substance to be toxic, and then decides to dump them, 'making surplus fat' to do so.

In the conventional treatment of allergic reactions the drug route can once more be implicated in PFR. Most of the drugs used to treat allergies are known to cause weight gain in some who take them, although this may not tip over into PFR. The most effective, and the most dangerous, drugs used for allergy treatment are steroids. Long-term use can produce a characteristic accumulation of fat in the 'dowager's hump' on the upper back. Fat is also laid down on the trunk and the face; those who take steroids for long periods are characterized by their round 'moon' faces.

Antihistamines, the most commonly used drugs for allergic problems, can induce weight gain. They may also have the effect of depressing the immune system, thus making some people more vulnerable to both infections and toxins. Some of the new types, free from the side-effect of drowsiness common with the older forms, have nevertheless been observed to cause weight gain in some users.

Our conclusion is that anyone who is susceptible to allergic reactions is at an increased risk of developing PFR. Such a person's system is juggling at various levels with substances it does not like; what action it will take if it should fail, or if it has to cope with more, is unpredictable, but PFR is an obvious long-stop.

We have now to consider the wider causes of PFR, the sources of overload of the systems we have been discussing. Drugs which our bodies treat as toxic are taken usually through choice, and we can control this source. But we are all taking in substances, both acknowledged poisons and others considered 'safe', all the time. We are all to some degree poisoned without being aware of it.

Everyone in the Western world now carries some poisoned fat on their body. Indeed, it may be true that everyone in the world is contaminated. This is because the sort of substances which migrate easily into fat are everywhere in our environment. The example of DDT illustrates how they can affect us.

DDT (dichlorodiphenyltrichloroethane) is, or rather was, a highly effective pesticide. It was widely used against everything from body lice and flies to mosquitoes in country-wide anti-malarial campaigns. Over the last four decades millions of tons have been released into the environment. The chemical is very bio-specific – it tends to attach itself to living organisms – and lethal to many pest species . . . until they acquire immunity.

The problem is that DDT is not biodegradable. In fact, it is rather the opposite, a molecule which combines its bio-specific qualities with a very high motivation, working hard to incorporate itself into living matter. It is almost as if it were working its way up the food chain, away from those insects which are now immune to it, into more complex animals which find it more difficult to deal with. Could this molecule's aim be to become an essential component of living cells? This idea is not really fantastic; all the organic molecules now incorporated in the life-forms of our biosphere must have moved up in this way during the evolution of life. The question at the back of our minds should be, how many of the thousands of bio-specific molecules we now use have the same properties?

Studies of the chemical composition of human fat reveal that all of us carry residues of DDT, dieldrin and other persistent organic insecticides. These were once used with what amounted to gay abandon – they still are in some parts of the world.

Our tissues are also saturated with metabolites of additives from food, those ubiquitous E substances. Preservatives, for example, do not only preserve the meat we eat; they also linger in our flesh with the same effect. Both American and British undertakers have reported that corpses actually stay fresh for two to three weeks longer than they used to!

We take in these substances with our food, in the air we breathe, and we absorb them through our skin. Exactly what happens to them depends on our individual metabolism, susceptibility and the nature and quantity of the substances to which we are exposed. Different forms of potential poison also interact with one another to complicate further any predictions we might try to make about their effects.

This hideous complexity effectively means that we are gambling with our bodies all the time. We cannot hope to predict or understand completely all that is going on. Nevertheless, some general principles are quite clear. Fat deposition is most likely to occur when we are exposed to substances our bodies treat as poisonous, and these substances are readily soluble in fat.

The most important of these are organic compounds based on carbon ring systems. All life on this planet is based on molecules assembled around carbon atoms, and the artificial molecules manufactured by industrial chemists are based on the hydrocarbon ring systems found in oil and coal – this is why such products are termed 'organic'. The substances produced around these molecular rings are few in nature, but our synthetic world is full of them. The register of artificial substances lists over seven million.

Everyday solvents such as formaldehyde, alcohol and other more complex substances such as those used for dry cleaning are also likely to end up in our fat – though often not in their original form. The real problem with these substances is their characteristic ability to precipitate liver damage with intensive short-term exposure or, in some cases, with long-term low-dose exposure, and it is this that the body seeks to avoid by dumping them in fat. So we have the additional possibility of substances causing liver damage, thus helping other substances to gain access to our tissues.

At the core of the cause of each victim's PFR is the capacity of the liver to respond to the demands placed upon it by the avalanche of substances loaded on to the system. If the liver is damaged or short of essential detoxifying agents, then the body's detoxification system may be greatly reduced. People whose livers are not functioning properly are bound to be more susceptible to the accumulation of toxic adiposity and the PFR Syndrome. This is because there is less capacity than when it works at peak efficiency.

Such PFR victims include individuals who have suffered damage due to drugs, chemicals or alcohol, as well as those who have had hepatitis (which means liver inflammation and has a variety of causes), malaria, Weil's disease, amoebic dysentry, bilharzia or allergic liver disease. And it will also include some of those who have difficulties in food absorption, or who are undernourished for any reason.

Many PFR sufferers will not realize that their livers are less efficient than normal. But some will know that they cannot tolerate more than a very small quantity of alcohol, or that they had a bad reaction to a hospital anaesthetic, or that they have a tendency to get unwell periodically, suffering nausea, indigestion and headaches.

Clinical ecologists, working in the field of allergic responses, have identified what they term 'subclinical malaise'. This is that vague feeling of being one or two degrees under, not up to much most of the time. This very widespread reaction is believed to be due to overload by low-level environmental toxins. It may not be enough to trigger PFR in most people, but it should be taken as a warning of possible susceptibility.

While acute liver disease is fairly readily diagnosed by the jaundice that results, producing a yellow colour in the skin as bile salts build up in the blood, the symptoms of chronic liver disease are vague. Sufferers feel generally unwell. Many have indigestion and some lose weight because the liver plays a crucial role in the digestion of food. In many cases, the liver does not come under suspicion for a long time – if at all.

There are chemical tests of liver function, but these are rather hit-and-miss; most can produce entirely normal results while disturbances in other crucial enzyme systems go undetected. And even if the liver copes quite well much of the time, a slightly increased load on its detoxification capacity will mean that the protective system that produces fat deposition will come into play.

The whole question of the possible causes of PFR may seem impossibly grim and we would not wish to diminish the size of the environmental problem that PFR represents. But once you understand how the systems concerned work, you will see how it is possible to work to overcome both cause and effects.

CHAPTER 7

PFR – The Theoretical Model

In this chapter we shall consider some theoretical aspects of persistent fat retention. If this is not your immediate interest, go on to page 61, and pick this up later.

You may find some of the concepts difficult to grasp at first. Although we have endeavoured to explain each step, many of the ideas may be unfamiliar. You do not need this knowledge to overcome your PFR problem. However, we believe that understanding its nature in some detail could help you to fit the escape strategy described in subsequent chapters more precisely to your personal needs.

To understand the mechanism involved in PFR we have to take a broad look at liver functions. The liver is little short of awe-inspiring. It is the most marvellous organ, the largest gland in the body and in many ways the most complicated. It carries out twenty-two known major functions, ranging from the digestion and storage of food, the synthesis of body constituents and the regulation of the chemical balance of the blood, to temperature control.

The liver lies on the right-hand side of the body behind the ribs, just under the diaphragm. It is closely interconnected with the heart and the nervous system at many levels. It is linked to the small intestine by a special vein (the hepatic portal vein), which carries food constituents absorbed through the lining of the gut.

The liver secretes bile which pours out through the bile duct into the duodenum just below the stomach. Bile plays a crucial role in fat digestion. Most of the bile is reabsorbed by the gut and recycled by the liver, very little being lost in the process.

Blood, rich in digestive products and the assortment of chemicals that we take in with our food and drink, circulates through six-sided 'liver lobules', where the complicated processes of biotransformation take place. Liver cells are very similar to one another, each one a highly sophisticated organ. Chemicals which enter are modified in a wide variety of ways by the host of enzyme systems which each cell contains.

Protein synthesis is one of the jobs done by the liver lobule cells. In the gut, food is broken down so that proteins arrive in the liver in the form of amino acids, the building blocks of all living tissue. The enzyme systems of the liver take these amino acids and reassemble them into proteins that are useful to us. These are then secreted into an exit vein that carries them to the heart, which pumps them round the rest of the body.

Carbohydrate foodstuffs are digested so that they arrive at the liver as glucose. The liver cells then build some of this into a long-chain simple carbohydrate called glycogen. Glycogen is stored in the liver itself, from where it can be quickly mobilized to provide energy when necessary, for instance to fuel a burst of physical activity. If you suddenly have to sprint to escape from a predator, or if you decide to do a bout of any strenuous activity, the local store of fuel in your muscles will run out very quickly. It is replenished by glycogen from the liver, which is broken down into glucose again and released into the bloodstream under the influence of the flight-or-fight hormone, adrenalin.

In men, the liver's glycogen store is very large. It evolved under conditions of life in our hunting and gathering past, when men were the hunters. Women have much smaller glycogen stores in livers which are smaller both in absolute terms and in relation to their total body size. They have evolved different fuelling systems to suit their gatherer and maternal role. Their bodies tend to run on current-account energy and to store fuel in the more slowly released but longer lasting form of fat, principally in that troublesome subcutaneous layer.

As well as for energy, the liver acts as a store for certain vitamins and minerals. It is generally known that liver can be an excellent type of food; this is mainly because it is so rich in the stored vitamins A, B group and D, as well as iron and zinc. The role of the liver in digestion, storage and release of nutrients into the rest of the body, is the reason we described it earlier as a vast marshalling yard; as you will now realize, it is also the body's prime industrial area. From this power base it regulates metabolism throughout the rest of the body. The nervous and hormone systems provide feedback loops which allow this regulation to occur. However, it is not a one-way process – the liver responds to needs, as well as directing them.

Any body product that is available for recycling will also go through the liver. Every part of our body is constantly being used, broken down and replaced. It is a part of that process of homeostasis mentioned in chapter 2. The products of breakdown reach the liver, where they are either sent off for excretion or reused. One example is bile pigments, which are actually made by the liver from the debris of red blood corpuscles.

This is another reason for the development of detoxifying capacity in the liver. Some products of normal metabolism are themselves toxic. Some parts of the body, such as the intestine, produce ammonia, which is poisonous in more than very small concentrations. The liver lobules change ammonia into urea, which can then be eliminated, via the kidneys, in urine.

The crucial and more complicated issue here is the role of the liver in the conversion of chemicals foreign to our bodies, including those of natural origin, but more especially of foreign artificial substances produced by man.

During evolution, which produced our sexually differentiated livers and their relatively different metabolisms working under the influence of different hormone mixtures, we encountered environmental toxins. These were toxins in plants and fungal byproducts, as well as those produced by bacteria. Some of these can still occur in the human diet, especially in the tropics. The metabolic systems that our ancestors developed to break them down are the same ones that now have to cope with the massive chemical load to which we are daily exposed. This load consists of tens of thousands of entirely artificial substances.

The substances that end up in our bloodstream are dealt with in those liver lobule cells that are already busy handling digestion and recycling nutrients. To carry out this work each liver cell relies on a sort of sub-cell within it, the mitochondrion. Mitochondria are sausage-shaped structures, consisting of libraries of hundreds of enzymes designed to deal with any substance they may encounter. There may be many mito-chondria in each liver cell. Each cell in the body has mitochon-dria; thus a molecular message sent out by the liver can be reinterpreted by reference to a similar library of enzyme in-formation when it reaches its destination.

One enzyme system in the liver cell mitochondria is known as Cytochrome P-450 (CP 450). There are, in fact, a number of CP 450s. At first it was assumed that just one enzyme had the particular characteristics that identified this class but, as with vitamins and many other chemical components of our incredibly complicated bodies, further research is constantly revealing more forms.

CP 450s are capable of bringing about a range of oxidative chemical reactions. Specifically, this means they can cause a poison or drug molecule to react with oxygen, and while CP 450s must be present for this to occur, they are left unchanged at the end of the reaction. Other chemical substances, both complex organic molecules and minerals including iron, are also involved but, like the cytochromes, while they must be present for the reaction to occur, they are not actually used up in the process.

This is the first stage of metabolism of such substances. The rate at which it occurs depends on the availability of appropriate CP 450s and on oxygen from the air we breathe. This stage is blocked by carbon monoxide – which is present in the blood of smokers in a concentration which is directly proportional to the number of cigarettes they smoke.

Because there are many CP 450s acting as catalysts for a range of different reactions, there can be many products of this first stage of metabolism. Each drug or toxin can in fact be altered in a lot of different ways. The problem is that these products of first-stage CP 450 reactions are often more poisonous than the original substance. This is because they have been made more chemically reactive by the addition of oxygen, and another step in metabolism must follow quickly to deal with this hazard.

This second stage of toxin metabolism usually involves a substance called glutathione. This joins on to the reactive intermediate and alters it so that it is no longer so dangerous to the body. However, glutathione is in limited supply, so sometimes this second stage of metabolism cannot keep pace with the production of highly reactive poisons by the CP 450 system. Under these circumstances, the liver – and the rest of the body – can get poisoned.

This problem of the increased reactivity of oxidized metabolic products, and their frequently dangerous nature, plus the apparently illogical shortage of glutathione, is a hangover from the very distant past. It is a reminder that to life on this planet at one time, oxygen was a highly poisonous substance. Most cellular components are still protected from it; they function anaerobically, that is, in the absence of oxygen. Aerobic activity occurs at a series of progressively restricted sites, from our lungs, through our bloodstream, to those actual cellular reactions that require oxygen for the release of chemical energy.

The dangers of the shortage of glutathione can be illustrated by what can happen when someone takes an overdose of paracetamol (acetaminophen). The CP 450s add oxygen to the basically fairly innocuous paracetamol molecule – and make it into a very dangerous substance. If there is not enough glutathione available in the liver to complete the second stage of metabolism, liver damage results. Death from liver failure occurs days or even weeks after the overdose.

Obviously, the body has ways of coping with slight

imbalances. In most biological reactions, the rate at which the first one or two stages of a sequence occurs depends partly on the rate at which subsequent steps are occurring. There are systems of feedback which allow the processes to be self-limiting and safe. But the picture can be complicated by the effects of certain chemical substances on the CP 450 system itself.

The effect of many products developed by the chemical industry is to interfere with the checks and balances in this crucial detoxification system. Drugs such as barbiturates, many pesticides, certain industrial chemicals and components of cigarette smoke, are capable of speeding up the CP 450s. They can induce the creation of higher concentrations of certain CP 450s, and thus cause the reactions to occur preferentially. The result can be a range of strange and dangerous intermediates produced at a higher than normal rate.

Such intermediates have been linked with cancer. The ability of cigarette smoke to alter the detoxification systems of the liver in this way could account for the fact that smoking is associated with cancers in many parts of the body where the smoke itself never goes. These include cancer of the liver itself, and of the cervix, bladder, pancreas and other organs.

One general class of compounds which are recognized to speed up the CP 450 system is called 'polycyclic hydrocarbons'. What this means is that they are compounds which have two or more rings of carbon molecules in them. Artificial substances with this type of molecular structure are very common products in our industrialized culture.

We spray millions of gallons of polycyclic hydrocarbon insecticides every year, but because we are not dying like flies or other 'bugs' we would be foolish to imagine we can escape without any harmful effect. The human body has a marvellous ability to resist the effects of potentially lethal chemicals, but they have to compete for the limited resources of the detoxifying enzyme systems. These systems are linked up with other biochemical processes in our bodies, and thus a further range of secondary effects may be generated.

The CP 450s are important, for example, in the metabolism of hormones. Sex hormones and steroids, both of which occur naturally and are also produced in synthetic forms for therapy, are structurally related to polycyclic hydrocarbons. As such they will be broken down in the same sort of way. So altering the balance of metabolic pathways could have implications for our body's response to its own hormones.

The questions we are raising here concern the way different organic substances interact with one another. These interactions involve both natural and artificial products: those that originate within the body and those we take in from outside. One documented area of interaction is through induction of the CP 450 system. One general consequence is likely to be a state of overload in the second stage of detoxification. Others, including competition for transport systems, are known; more undoubtedly exist but are as yet unidentified.

PFR involves transporting unwanted and potentially dangerous substances into storage organs where they will do little damage. For organic compounds of the type we have been discussing, the store is fat. Most are readily dissolved in fat and can stay there in a reasonably stable state for as long as necessary.

Potentially dangerous chemicals are not normally allowed to float around freely in the bloodstream. They are attached for transport from one place to another to special carriers. In the liver, these substances are known as 'ligandins': we think of them as biological wheelbarrows. Again there can be competition between different metabolic products for these wheelbarrows; many can be moved by the same ligandin, but the availability may be limited – like taxis on rainy days.

Once at a suitable deposit point, in this case a fat cell, the carrier will release its toxic load into solution in the fatty interior. This is only possible if the concentration of chemicals already in solution in the fat is not too high. For the dumping system to work at its best, the body may need to add fat to the cells to increase their volume and thus to reduce the concentration of toxins within.

Obviously, this protective mechanism is itself finely balanced. The liver must be working effectively enough to make fat available to pump up the fat cells in order to cushion the effects of poisons. Your body must have an adequate quantity of fat cells and the systems for filling them must function fast and efficiently. And there must be sufficient calories in the diet to allow the deposition of fat.

If these conditions are not met when the liver is overloaded or stimulated into producing poisonous metabolites of the chemicals it processes, then the effects of the poisons will be much worse. Instead of getting fat, you are likely to get ill.

When the capacity of the liver to adapt and use different metabolic pathways is limited by poisons or disease, then it may not be capable of dealing with chemicals in this way. In some conditions, such as cirrhosis due to alcohol, it has been observed that sufferers can be quite obese in the early stages of the disease, when the overloaded liver is shifting toxins into fat. Then, as the condition progresses and the liver becomes less and less capable of functioning normally, they start to waste away.

This, then, is how poisons can make you fat. Because of the body's need to protect itself, it will set up and give priority to this complete chain of reactions. This is the metabolic basis of the Persistent Fat Retention Syndrome.

Once the metabolism has established this mechanism, its preferential use will tend to be established. Preferentiality may produce some addictive reaction to the substances that body treats in this way. The system comes to anticipate the loading they provide, and behaves disruptively if this anticipation is not fulfilled.

Stores of fat saturated with toxins are what we have called toxic adipose tissue. Its status is constantly monitored by the body, and especially by the central chemical control centre, the liver. Fat is a relatively stable store because it is not involved in active metabolic processes most of the time and it does not have a plentiful blood supply, but it is nevertheless kept in equilibrium with the general chemical balance of the body. If the blood is loaded with poisons but the fat cells are relatively free of them, then more will be dumped; but if the blood is clear of them, then they will tend to be picked up from contaminated fat to be dealt with by the liver.

If the liver successfully completes its metabolic sequence, unwanted chemicals can finally be eliminated from the body. The most used route is via the kidneys, which filter water-soluble products from the blood. Even at this stage, some of these substances may still be poisonous. While they are bound to their biological carriers in the blood they do no damage; but when they leave them in the tubules of the kidneys they are capable, once more, of causing injury. And many drugs and chemicals are known to poison liver and kidney alike.

We have referred so far mainly to recognized poisons, for it is the metabolism of these that has been studied by toxicologists. But what your body treats as poisonous will not be just those chemicals that are known to poison everybody. You may react to a wide range of normally harmless substances as though they were poisonous because your body has mis-identified them. This is the basis of allergy, and it can form a separate route into PFR for those susceptible.

In the context of a heavy environmental loading of artificial substances which have a high affinity with our natural processes, problems are bound to arise. The systems concerned will be chronically overloaded, and this is exactly what precipitates allergic responses. An allergy is a changed response to a stimulus; more usually it is thought of as an exaggerated and inappropriate response to a food or other substance.

In our case histories we outlined an example of one person, predisposed to allergic responses, who subsequently developed a cyclical PFR response to his allergic condition. The allergic route into PFR is less clear than the mechanism of detoxification overload detailed above; nevertheless, some features can be sketched in.

Allergic reactions of all sorts are increasing. The common

condition, hay fever, now affects between ten and fifteen per cent of the population in every industrialized nation. Hay fever was unknown two hundred years ago. The first recorded victims were doctors, who had difficulty finding other sufferers. Its growth to a condition which annually afflicts millions runs exactly parallel to the growth of industrialization; doctors may have been the first victims because they used to mix their own medicines, many of which were new chemical compounds. Hay fever offers further confirmation that we cannot expose ourselves, or our environment, to *ad lib* pollution without adversely affecting our health.

We believe that many of the emerging allergic reactions, particularly to food, are caused by the same pollution which leads to PFR and conditions such as hay fever. They may be attributed to the residues of pesticide sprays and processing chemicals, molecules of which can be found in almost all of our food. A wider base of allergic response may be generated by carbon-based molecules in our general environment, and underwritten by the old-fashioned 'lump and rubbish' pollution which we now all accept as undesirable.

Allergic reactions are generated by the body's immune systems. These are complex interactive systems, working at every level within the body, designed to protect it against the effects of foreign invaders and functional errors like the production of cancer cells. To carry out its protective function the immune system has to be able to identify a vast range of molecules and life forms. To do this it has libraries of information to which it can refer; we add to one part of this information bank when we become immune to a particular disease. The profile of the disease entity is registered and antibodies are developed to counter it.

Disease entities are, in general, fairly large and distinct organisms. Our immune system works on the basis of recognition of the protein pattern of their outer coating. It also has to be capable of much finer recognition, down to the molecular level. In hay fever sufferers, pollen grains mistaken for pathogens cause mast cells to degranulate. This degranulation releases a flood of unpleasant chemicals, including histamine, intended to make life unpleasant or impossible for the supposedly dangerous invader. While mast cells remain intact, it is thought that their crystalline structure is analogous to a memory chip, assessing the food and other molecules which constantly pass their strategic sites in the body.

The number of carbon-based artificial molecules now present in our environment overload these systems, and it only takes a pollen grain to trigger a totally inappropriate response. The whole immune system is a complex and finely balanced system. Like all such systems the degree to which their function can be stretched without breakdown occurring will be limited.

The liver is the final destination for much of the debris produced by the work of the immune systems. The chemical and biological warfare with which the systems respond to perceived threats places a load on the liver. Normally this poses no problem; these systems are working all the time, usually we are completely unaware of it. Only when we become ill, through a temporary failure or extended battle with an infection, is it brought to our attention. Nevertheless, in susceptible individuals, it is quite feasible that the strain of allergic overload could substantially reduce detoxification capacity for toxins arriving from other sources. In such cases PFR is a possible and perhaps common outcome.

The general danger of all the pesticide residues to which we are exposed is that they are capable of affecting almost any level of our being. These substances are designed to work by disrupting the life-form at which they are aimed. They do this principally by punching holes in cell membranes, thereby destroying the integrity of the cell and killing it.

This mechanism has been used for our benefit in the past; it is the way penicillin works. The penicillin molecule becomes incorporated in the bacterial cell during its growth and disrupts the integrity of the structure, making it non-viable. However, as we know, many bacteria have acquired resistance to penicillin;

they have done this by learning to take the penicillin molecule apart, rendering it ineffective. Sooner or later, most pest species acquire resistance to the pesticides used against them. Indeed, some seem to bounce back with renewed vigour: the salmonella bacterium, an increasing problem for hospitals and the general population, is one such example. It is a growing problem because of the regular dosing of factory-farmed animals with antibiotics, which renders these drugs ineffective when used against human infections. Another example is the super-rat, which now thrives on the warfarin put out as poison.

As the pesticides become more refined, so they are deployed against more specialized systems within the target organism; but in their turn, these more specialized systems have greater capacity to achieve resistance. Thus a never-ending circle, highly profitable for pesticide manufacturers, is created.

For humans, problems may be accentuated by the fact that our cell membranes are made principally of fatty substances, especially cholesterol. The possible problems caused by the affinity of pesticide for fats become at this point almost infinite.

The organophosphates, the pesticides which now predominate in modern farming, are said to be non-persistent. We have, however, been able to find no convincing explanation of their final biodegradability into harmless products in our environment. We suspect that their use is encouraged by a general belief that they simply go away. Because of this, those bodies charged with investigating residue problems do not tend to look for these substances or their breakdown products, concentrating instead on less used insecticides. Many of the breakdown products of pesticides are not even known, and will therefore not be found by the methods of analysis now used. This leaves wide open the possibilities of adverse effects of the widespread use of such substances.

CHAPTER 8

Are You What You Eat?

Most of us grew up with the assumption that we could eat anything, in any quantity, without coming to any real harm. We accepted that if it was on the shelf, it would be safe.

It was only very recently that the dangers of relying on industrially manufactured fast foods were recognized. The malnutrition among plenty caused by junk foods led to some questioning of this underlying assumption. Dieters discovered the problem of the empty calorie – enticing junk which caused nutritional problems.

Behind consumer awareness campaigns came the declaration that 'you are what you eat', implying that if you relied on junk to feed and maintain you, you would turn into unhealthy junk. Many of us now accept the wisdom of avoiding junk food, although it is regrettably true that the profits of such enterprises continue to grow.

The idea that has always been pushed by dieticians and nutrition experts is that of the balanced diet. What this usually amounts to is this; if your diet contains sufficient variety of foods, with an emphasis on fresh fruit and vegetables, is not short of protein, natural vitamins and trace elements, you will be all right. Unfortunately, as the health statistics in general and those for obesity specifically show, either we have ignored this advice or it is incorrect.

While many do ignore the basic commonsense of such an approach to food, we believe that the ill-health associated with food is out of all proportion to the imbalances in our national diet. The PFR Syndrome is part of this imbalance; many Life Profile cases had eating habits beyond reproach. We believe the possibility exists that a mountain of other specific conditions, as well as a groundswell of minor incapacitation, can be directly traced to what we are doing to our food.

While we have become aware of the health hazards of fast-food, we have been slow to react to other changes that have occurred over the past few decades. The whole food industry has been subjected to one of the most profound revolutions the world has ever experienced. But because of the strength of that assumption – if it's on the shelf it must be safe – we have scarcely noticed what has been happening. We have all heard of the green revolution, but that was just a public relations smoke-screen covering the reality of what was happening to our food.

Other factors have helped to mask the profound changes which have been going on. One is the depopulation of the countryside; the majority of people are no longer involved in food production, whereas only a generation or so ago the reverse was true. We knew about the quality of food from direct personal experience; we were not fooled by the packaging as we are now. Another factor is our general omnivorous nature; we can eat almost anything, and survive if not thrive on it. This capacity has coloured our attitude to food; it has advantages but also drawbacks. It may have led us into complacent acceptance of things we should forcefully reject.

Our food has always been a source of potentially toxic substances. Indeed, it was probably exposure to this risk throughout our evolution that led to the development of the liver's detoxifying capacity. Through surviving the effects of poisonous plants and fruits, we learned to avoid them.

Where sources of toxins were obvious, as with the leaves of potato or rhubarb, or the brightly coloured berries of night-shade or laburnum, avoiding eating them was straightforward. But nature is not always so obvious. Many fungi contain poisons; not only the toadstools which cause confusion among the wild mushrooms, but also those microscopic varieties which make foods mouldy. If you cannot see them, it may be difficult to avoid being poisoned.

Through the work of people like Pasteur, remembered in the way we make milk safe, this microsphere of life was uncovered and further avoiding action taken. It is still true that invisible natural poisons kill many people in less developed parts of the world today; moulds which grow on peanuts under warm damp conditions of tropical regions cause thousands of deaths from liver cancer in those parts of the world. Some of these fungal poisons have been found to have uses; ergot, which grows on rye and used to cause a wide range of bizarre and finally fatal effects in those who ate a critical dose, now yields the anti-migraine drug ergotamine. By and large, however, our ancestors would have found out by trial and error which foods were contaminated with invisible toxins. The capacity to survive mild poisoning was obviously an advantage; otherwise the lesson would have to be learned anew by each generation.

Why is it so difficult to get wholesome food today? The simple answer is because of the food industry. Each part of the chain, from farmer to shopkeeper, has forgotten what it is supposed to be doing: supplying the consumer with safe, wholesome produce. Farmers, who used to have a hard, healthy life in the great outdoors, are now agribusinessmen prone to heart disease and extracting annual returns from sterile green deserts. And those grocers who once characterized our nation, whose shops and wares could be judged by eye, are now insulated by plastic wrapping and corporate structures from the reality of their goods.

Today the invisible poisons we confront are no longer provided by nature; they are man-made. They are added to our food chains continually, from before birth or planting, throughout growth, during harvesting and storage, through all the subsequent processing to the moment we eat the final product.

The residues of pesticides can be found in most foods, even the fish caught in the open sea far from farm and factory.

Processing additives are put into food for a variety of reasons and often consumers are persuaded to add their own dash of adulteration. All of these chemicals are of course considered 'safe' by the relevant government institutions we assume are watching our interests in this area. But is this in fact the case? Mounting evidence points to an emphatic 'No!'

We accept that each of the substances involved, in a low concentration, may be safe for the majority of people. And also that many people will be able to cope with a diet which contains many such substances. But we can only describe as very fortunate those who have bodies efficient enough to cope, day after day, with the assault that the modern food industry delivers.

The fact is that as this assault grows in intensity and complexity, fewer and fewer people are able to cope. As our chemical loading grows with the progressive industrialization of food production, our protective systems are forced to work harder. Each new molecule has to be identified and decisions taken about how it should be dealt with. The systems in our body which do this are finely tuned, evolved to manage threats which developed relatively slowly in our biosphere, and they were very good at this. Asking them to cope with tens of thousands of totally artificial substances is like trying to use a violin as a cricket bat; eventual breakdown is inevitable.

As manufacturers seek to extend the shelf-life and profitability of food, more additives are used. It is these substances which cause the greatest problem for many people. In general terms, food which is high in additives is low in nutrition. Consuming such foods is a part of the degenerative cycle which can lead to PFR; your systems have to work harder to deal with them, for a lower reward. Of course this has led to the suggestion that slimmers could eat a lot of non-nutritional substances, thus feeling full without putting on weight. This is near the ultimate in using your body as a dustbin – treat it like one and it will look like one. It is likely to have exactly the opposite effect on your weight from that which you wanted.

You probably believe that somewhere, someone is in control of the question of food additive safety. In theory, the use of food additives is controlled by the Food and Drugs Act 1955. This Act requires that additives be kept to a minimum, and any new additive must be shown to be 'technologically essential as well as safe'. The facts of their use, however, make a mockery of such parliamentary gentility. Such exhortations are rather like asking a bank robber to observe the provisions of the highway code during his getaway.

Today there are about 3,500 different food additives in use; no one is sure exactly how many. In the last decade alone the quantities used have doubled. They are in such widespread use that on average everyone consumes eleven pounds of food additives each year. The food industry spent in excess of £160m on them in 1984.

There are also around 3,000 food flavourings. These, along with starches and enzymes, are barely regulated at all. Precisely what many of them are is considered to be a commercial secret. A raspberry flavouring for a food product that has to withstand high temperatures and pressures during manufacture may contain seven or more flavouring chemicals. The only people who know what these are work for the company that makes the product.

While there is a growing wave of public concern about the whole question of additives, the government is not impressed. At the last count the appropriate body was regulating the use of just 314 substances, less than ten per cent of those used. As we shall see, public concern may be justified if only on the grounds that Britain, as frequently happens, allows substances to go into our food that have been banned elsewhere.

As consumers, we are generally led to believe that food additives would not be permitted if they had not been proved safe. But what little toxicity testing there is cannot be trusted to protect us from the potential hazards of these chemicals. Dr Eric Millstone of Sussex University reports that the Director of the British Industrial Biological Research Association (BIBRA) has admitted that 'food additive toxicology is . . . merely a technology designed to produce animal test data sufficient to gain permission from governments for the use of additives.' Further, it 'is not a science which seeks to understand the biological effects of chemicals upon humans.'

As if this were not bad enough, the reality of use of these chemicals is totally discounted. The tests that are carried out by toxicologists ignore the fact that we are exposed to a great number of these substances at once. One particular food product may contain as many as thirty different additives, but they are never tested in combination.

Nor can we rely on the animal tests that are carried out to discover long-term effects of humans. The study of drug effects has shown that reactions are frequently 'species specific'. This means that a food additive which has no effect on mice could be disastrous to humans, because although there are many similarities, mice and men are different species. Then, if this additive in use caused serious damage to one person in a thousand who consumed it, and minor damage to one in every hundred, we might never know. Epidemiology, the recording of diseases among whole populations, would be most unlikely to reveal the problem before it reached enormous proportions. Think about cigarettes: they kill one in four of lifetime smokers, yet they were not identified as dangerous for over a quarter of a century.

The food additive minefield is in many ways like prescription drugs before thalidomide. Everyone assumes that all is well, everyone trusts the other person to behave reasonably, and the momentum of the past keeps the system going. It is only when some disaster occurs that any heed is taken of warnings. It is unlikely that food additives will produce a watershed tragedy like thalidomide. Nevertheless, it must be acknowledged that the load these substances place on the population as a whole is responsible for a slow moving wave of illness and malaise which is inevitably growing as time goes by. Slowly developing phenomena always take time to recognize, and even once their source and nature is recognized, such large, slow waves take a long time to stop.

Some food additives are already known to produce illness in a disturbingly large proportion of people. The best documented example is E102, tartrazine, a yellow colouring. In *E for Additives*, Professor Maurice Hanssen describes tartrazine as 'a very commonly used colour'. It can cause skin rashes, hay fever (paradoxically, it was used to colour antihistamine tablets), breathing problems, blurred vision, gastric upsets and purple blotches on the skin. Just how many people are susceptible to any of these effects is a matter of wide controversy; estimates range from less than 1 per cent to over 20 per cent of the population.

Naturally, the food industry argues that such risks are minimal. And they are supported by the Royal College of Physicians of London, who produced a Joint Report on Food Intolerance in 1984 with the food-industry-funded British Nutrition Foundation. Under Sir Douglas Black (who also produced the government's reassuring report on the high incidence of leukaemia near Sellafield) a press conference was held to counter what was described as public 'hysteria' about food allergies. Careful reading of their report, however, revealed the admission that 'no estimate can be made of the prevalence of food intolerance because of a lack of adequate information. With the exception of rare but specific biochemical effects, diagnostic methods . . . are highly subjective.'

Some readers may find it distressing that such an eminent body could pronounce emphatically on a phenomenon which could not be measured because of a lack of adequate information. But doctors are, after all, only human, and subject to the same prejudices as the rest of us. Perhaps we could expect more discretion in their expression. It may come as no surprise to learn that similarly eminent medical practitioners could be found to swear on oath that thalidomide did not, in their opinion, cause the birth defects attributed to it.

Tartrazine is one of a group of related food colours, (E104-110; E122-133) the azo dyes, which are derived from coal tar. All have been implicated in hyperactivity, and some, such as red E123, amaranth, have been linked with birth defects in animals. Amaranth has been banned in the United States.

Some of the most dangerous of the additives used in Britain are the butylate antioxidants, E320 and E321. They are added to fats to prevent rancidity, and may be found in margarine, vegetable oils and many baked products containing fat. They have been linked with allergic reactions and liver problems. Government reports have twice recommended that they be restricted and they are not permitted in baby foods, yet they are the most widely used antioxidants in this country.

The benzoates (numbers E210 to E219) are preservatives and mould retardants. Benzoyl peroxide is used to bleach flour. These chemicals are known to be hazardous to allergy sufferers and have been restricted in the USSR because they cause brain damage and convulsions, and retard growth in animals.

The nitrates (E250 to E252) are also used as preservatives. It is these which give the pink colour to meat products. Nitrates are broken down to nitrites in the body and, to some degree, during cooking. These interact with amines from food and drugs to produce nitrosamines – which are carcinogenic. These additives can also cause allergic reactions, are implicated in arthritis and may interfere with the ability of the liver to store vitamin A. They have been banned in Norway.

Sulphites (E220-7, E513) are preservatives, antioxidants and bleaches. They are to be found in the highest concentration on dried fruit – especially apricots and other brightly-coloured fruits, for they stop them turning brown. They are also used in wines, beer, fruit juices and purées, soft drinks, jam, dried vegetables and biscuits. They destroy vitamins B and E, may cause genetic mutations, and some people are allergic to them.

Glutamates (E621-3) are 'flavour enhancers'. The most used, and best known, is monosodium glutamate (MSG). This was found to be the cause of 'Chinese restaurant syndrome', an illness typified by headaches, nausea, dizziness and pains in the neck, which can occur after a meal heavy in MSG.

A list of E numbers, giving information on which you should avoid and which are believed to be safe, is given in Appendix 1. They are not all potentially hazardous; in fact, some are valuable components of our normal diet. For example, carotene, which is transformed into vitamin A in our bodies, is a natural yellow dye with no known adverse effects. It is E160(a), and is often added to margarine and cakes.

The moves towards improved food labelling are intended to help people who are worried about additives to identify foods which may cause them problems. While this is to be welcomed, additives are only part of the problem. They are the most obvious form of chemical contamination of our food, but they may not be the most dangerous. Pesticide residues in food are both more poisonous, and harder to identify.

For farmworkers, spraying land with noxious chemicals has become the most common task. Increases in cancer deaths, and birth defects among their children, reveal the effects of this change among this previously very healthy group of workers. The 'tramlines' left in fields by the spraying machinery are everywhere in lowland Britain. During spring and early summer places such as East Anglia should, in our opinion, be closed to the public as health hazards.

There is no effective control on pesticide use. Despite the highly toxic nature of the many substances involved, there is no legislation designed to provide even minimal levels of protection for the public. Maximum residue levels are fixed by the Ministry of Agriculture, Farming and Fisheries (MAFF) and we believe much greater effort should be made to detect produce that exceeds these limits. Producers are not prosecuted for selling food contaminated with pesticides.

In fact, the MAFF inspectors who travel the country checking produce for quality would tend to downgrade produce which is not sprayed. These inspectors are actually discouraged from sending produce for pesticide analysis. The complicated chemical analyses required to detect potentially hazardous residues are carried out on a minute proportion of the food we eat – and no action is taken when problems are detected. Against this background the rate of spraying increases yearly as farmers get more and more dependent on pesticides. A dangerous cycle has been set up. It started with the excessive use of artificial fertilizers; these gave improved crop yields and encouraged farmers to break the traditional mixture of arable and pastoral farming which maintained a continuing natural soil fertility. Having broken this cycle, farmers had little choice other than to fertilize; this reduced the natural resilience of both soil and crops, so they had to use pesticides to limit pests. These still further reduced the soil's resilience, so more pesticides have to be used . . . Today farming is little better than an extractive industry, drawing contaminated crops from dead soils.

Between 1979 and 1982, the crop area sprayed with insecticides in Britain doubled and the area treated with fungicides more than doubled – yet the total cropped area scarcely increased. Over ten per cent of winter wheat is sprayed ten or more times. Twenty per cent of onions get ten to fifteen applications. Hops were sprayed an average of twenty-three times in 1979, orchards and soft fruit seventeen times. In total between 97 per cent and 99 per cent of fresh fruit, cereals and vegetables are sprayed at least once. The excessive record must go to one lettuce crop which was found to have been sprayed forty-six times with four different pesticides.

Farmers spray more and more just to maintain a constant level of crop 'quality'. The reasons for this are well recognized and the result is described as the 'pesticide treadmill'. In addition to the decrease in natural soil fertility, intensive mechanized agriculture leads to increasing use of pesticides because the natural resistance of crops to pests is decreasing, while the pests' resistance to chemicals is increasing. At the same time, spraying kills the normal predators of pests so that the biological controls which used to operate become ineffective.

In the past, pest levels were kept down by crop rotation,

ploughing and a natural balance between species; varieties of crops were selected for their ability to resist pests, and the quality of the soil was kept high enough to allow them to grow strong so that pests did not attack them too readily. And if lettuces arrived in the shops with greenfly on them, cabbages with the odd caterpillar, apples with occasional worms, nobody worried too much – it was only natural, after all.

If there are no controls down on the farm, what about controls on the produce which we eat? Our old and very feeble friend, the Food and Drugs Act of 1955, is supposed to control pesticide residues in food. To this end it states that food must be fit for human consumption, and not injurious to health. Unfortunately, those charged with the duty of implementing the Act limit themselves to preventing contamination by bacteria. In 1981 only 338 food samples were checked for residues under the provisions of this Act, but 87,000 were analysed for microbiological contamination.

While salmonella and similar bacterial problems do present a health hazard, the risk is relatively small among healthy populations. The government, its legislation and the practices of those carrying out policy just have not kept up to date with the changing reality of the modern world.

If food additives are in a pre-thalidomide situation, what of pesticides? The best analogy is that of the situation beloved in Victorian melodrama, where the most poisonous substances, like arsenic, could be bought over the counter in the village chemists, no questions asked. Later, villains could be caught by examination of the poisons book – if they were not clever enough to forge a signature. As we shall see, the control even of substances acknowledged to be dangerous and supposedly banned is roughly in a pre-poisons-book stage.

The Institute of Public Analysts has attempted to assess the size of the pesticide residue problem, and the results of their surveys are deeply disturbing. The respected *Journal of the Association of Public Analysts* published a report of the analysis of 305 fruits and 178 vegetables. Thirty-four per cent were found to be contaminated. One in ten fruits and one in five vegetables were above the MAFF 'reporting limits'. The data clearly reveal that the more samples of any type of produce were analysed, the higher was the chance of finding residues. The only conclusion to be drawn is that nothing is definitely safe.

You may think that analysing only 305 fruits and 178 vegetables is no basis for any rational assessment of the state of the thousands of tons of such foods we eat. But the MAFF, our safeguard in these matters, seems quite satisfied with even smaller samples.

In the Ministry's surveys just 9 of each of 22 food groups are checked – a grand total of 198 items. That means that the MAFF tests something like one in every 3,000 million potatoes we eat, a similar proportion of fruit, one in every 600 million tomatoes, and equally meaningless proportions of other foods. Yet the farmers complain of too many controls, and in 1985 the Deputy Minister of Agriculture, Tom McGregor, stated that the government maintains 'constant vigilance' in its watch for possible pesticide residues in food!

If the minimal testing by the MAFF is worrying, the substances found by the public analysts give even greater cause for concern. Some were the particularly persistent and dangerous types which are not approved for use on food.

DDT has been banned for any use on crops in Britain – yet this and its close relative DDE was found on blackcurrants, strawberries and lettuce. Aldrin and dieldrin, persistent pesticides of the same chemical group as DDT, are not cleared for use on any food except potatoes grown in former pasture (a very small proportion of the crop) – yet they were found contaminating spring onions, mushrooms, tomatoes, watercress and courgettes.

DDT was the insecticide which gave rise to the situation described in Rachel Carson's classic, *Silent Spring*. It is banned or severely restricted in many countries around the world. This widespread condemnation is based on the serious health risks both to wildlife (DDT is responsible for the virtual extinction of herons and falcons, and many other birds in East Anglia and elsewhere) and to humans. It accumulates in fat and causes liver damage.

After the scare caused in the early 1960s by the realization of the hazards, it was generally assumed that the problem had been dealt with. Despite this, British farmers continue to use it. Over 80 per cent of brassica growers in the East Anglian fens admitted to an Open University researcher that they were still using DDT against caterpillars, long after official approval had been withdrawn because of the hazards of this chemical. A second survey by the Association of Public Analysts (unpublished at the time of writing) reveals that ten per cent of all food samples analysed contained DDT or closely related chemicals. English apples, cabbage, lettuce and mushrooms were contaminated. In 1985 unlimited DDT is still on sale to British farmers, even though in theory it has been withdrawn.

So far we have discussed processed foods and fruit and vegetables. The situation with meat products is, if anything, even more serious. In spite of growing resistance among consumers to the factory farming of animals, 99 per cent of the meat we eat is produced in this way.

Factory farming is so unnatural that it only works because the animals are continually drugged. This is done both to control diseases, which are endemic under such conditions, and to stimulate growth. The latter involves hormones and antibiotics administered in food, by injection or by implantation. Moreover, the waste products of some animals are fed to others, for example, the waste from factory-farmed chickens is fed to intensively reared pigs.

These animals treat these substances in exactly the same way that we do, they metabolize many of them into their flesh. In addition to the development of resistant strains of bacteria such as salmonella from the liberal use of antibiotics, which pose a direct risk to humans, the metabolized products of the chemical assault these animals have to withstand is passed on to us.

Aldrin, and its breakdown product dieldrin, have been

banned or severely restricted in many countries. Like DDT, these pesticides accumulate in fat, cause liver damage and are suspected of causing cancer. These dangerous chemicals are still being used in sheep dip by some farmers in Wales and Devon, although clearance for this use was officially withdrawn in 1969. Residues are found in fat from the animals.

The MAFF appears to assume that there is no real pesticide problem. There have been no prosecutions of farmers who persist in contaminating crops with uncleared or withdrawn pesticides because there is, as yet, no law in this respect, and the ministry does not therefore have the necessary 'teeth'. DDT itself has been withdrawn since 1984.

Many of the substances we have been discussing are powerful biocides. Their purpose is to kill living things. While they may not kill you, they will kill some part of you. It is in fighting a desperate battle to protect you that your body is driven to maintain those fat stores. The only way you can safely escape from PFR is to stop this battle. Stop loading your system with food which should be classed as unfit for human consumption.

Take the battle outside your body. Just as you should not treat it as a dustbin, neither should you allow it to be a battlefield. You are what you eat. If you eat poisoned or contaminated food, you will be poisoned and contaminated. If your body cannot cope with this, it will react adversely. One of the ways it can react is by making you fat.

CHAPTER 9

Escape PFR – The Plan

Having read this far, you will have a pretty good idea of the situation you are in. You know that persistent fat is the product of a unique interaction between your metabolism and the many substances you are exposed to in your food and your environment.

Escaping PFR probably seems like a daunting prospect. Being stuck with weight you do not want, caused by factors which may appear to be largely beyond your control, can seem like being caught in a trap. But do not despair – escape is possible!

What you need is a good plan and a cool head. We can provide the plan, you have to provide the personal qualities. Like all successful escape plans, it depends upon coordination, timing and the ability to understand what is happening to you as you work your way through. We warned that this book was for those who seriously wanted to lose that excess weight.

We would like you to read this and the following three chapters before you attempt to take any action. Having done this you will understand what is involved in the Plan. This is important because it provides an integrated strategy; each part must be used in order, and in the correct relationship with the other parts. You may find it helpful to make notes of things which particularly apply to you and your situation as you read through. There are also some initial steps you can take to get you ready to apply the Plan; these are noted in this chapter.

We must once more stress the importance of individual differences. Because no two people are identical and we all live different lives, no single answer will produce the same effect on all of us. An important part of the success of the Plan is this: as you work through it, you will be learning about yourself. You must use this knowledge to judge the emphasis you need to give to each part of the Plan; how important diet is to you, how much contamination you can tolerate, how fast your progress should be. In short, you must be in control.

You are the active ingredient in the Plan. Passive acceptance of other people's diets, food products and environmental pollution has contributed to your PFR Syndrome. Now you must be assertive, you must start to fight back and we shall point you in the right direction. The ultimate objective is to learn to live in a way that suits your system and capacities best.

You will need high motivation; we will take that for granted. And you will need a fair measure of faith. Not in us, or this book, but in yourself. You need to learn to trust the signals from your body, to be able to look at yourself realistically, and to interpret any ambiguous signals accurately. When you understand what is happening to you, and why, then you will be in control.

Before getting down to details of the Plan, we must deal with the most likely cause of possible failure to solve your PFR problem. You will fail if you do not care about yourself sufficiently. You have got to prepare yourself in the same way that performers and athletes do before a big event, because you have got a lot of barriers to break through in your escape. The reason PFR is so common is that it is a reflection of values in our society. You have got to care enough, and be strong enough, to start going against the grain. You are fighting for yourself. At first you may feel lonely and daunted; don't – there are many more like you out there on the same battle, you will make friends and allies!

You will say, of course, that the reason you want to lose weight and be slim and fit, is precisely because you do care about yourself. Our experience indicates, however, that a lot of people go in for dieting, and even exercise, because they do not care. They are using the dieting syndrome as a way of punishing or rejecting their essential selves. The whole question of female sexuality, its development against a generally repressive social background, and the addition of body fat, is such a minefield for developing young women that fat and guilt become closely associated. Punishing their metabolism is the modern form of mortification of the flesh.

As your initial step, try looking at yourself naked in a full length mirror. Turn round, check yourself out all over, and write down your feelings about what you see. What are your best features, and what could do with some improving effort? Your answers may indicate that you have to escape from some psychological traps before you can successfully tackle your PFR problem.

Our culture teaches women self-rejection, almost self-abasement. We want you to look at yourself and feel pride. A justifiable pride in what you are and what you can become. Reject shallow narcissism that tells you to paint it over or cover it up with fabric. Modesty, false or real, is a route to submission and rejection. Look at the real you frequently, and with growing honest pride in the wonder of your body and yourself. You and those around you will be much better for your changed attitude.

The way you look at yourself may also indicate other bits of psychological baggage that you just do not need. Do you have unrealistic expectations about yourself? Losing weight will not make you taller or shorter. Although your bone structure will change, this takes a long time, and does not significantly affect height or proportions. Be realistic about the importance of weight loss in your life. We have one Life Profile client who is keeping her fat because she uses it as a way of making her husband feel sorry for her, and thus maintains the 'helpless woman' role that is apparently important to their relationship. This is an extreme case, but had she been able to be honest at the outset she would have saved herself a lot of half-hearted effort.

This book is not about the psychological aspects of weight problems, but their importance should not be overlooked. If you have any doubts at all in this area, which may upset your motivation to escape, check this out. You could follow up with one of the books on the psychology of self-acceptance. We would recommend Susie Orbach's excellent *Fat is a Feminist Issue*.

So before you start, it is important to be sure of yourself and your motivation!

The Escape Plan was designed primarily to deal with the PFR Syndrome, but it is not a slimming regime in the normal sense. Conventional approaches do not work for people with toxic adipose tissue, because as the old joke has it, 'you can't get there from here.'

To deal with PFR you have to gear your systems up to higher levels of health and give your metabolism greater capacity. That is the way you can get there. Of course, the Plan will make you slimmer, that is its primary objective, but not without making you much healthier in the process.

You have taken the first step by looking at yourself. Now take the second, affirm your own unique value. Write in your note book, 'I am the most important thing in my life.' Write it until you believe it, and can act on that belief without a second thought.

An important part of your new self-appreciation is to understand this: if you are a PFR victim and have contaminated fat you would rather be without, then your body has been doing an excellent job in protecting you from pollutants in your environment. Acknowledge that, look on that fat with new and wiser eyes, perhaps even appreciate what those extra pounds may have saved you from. Now make up your mind that you will return the favour and protect your body. Start by deciding 'I am not a rubbish dump, and my body is not going to be treated like one.'

The Plan has three separate aspects. These interact to produce their effect, but they must be initiated one after another, so that effects build up and complement each other. We will outline them in the order you need to carry them out.

Detoxification
Until the level of whatever substances your system is treating as toxic is drastically reduced in your bloodstream and liver, your body will not be ready to allow its fat stores to shrink.

Increasing Metabolic Capacity
This means creating the conditions where your liver can rebuild itself. Fortunately, this process will start automatically as the stress imposed on it is reduced. The Plan is designed both to assist this process and to increase your liver's capacity to handle loads it may encounter in the future.

Mobilizing Fat
This is the final and crucial stage. It cannot be achieved until your liver has sufficient capacity to cope with the toxins stored in this tissue.

To ensure that this capacity is at its highest, all the actions undertaken in the first two stages must be maintained throughout the third.

Warning: Losing toxic adiposity in any other way can cause serious illness. You will be releasing poisons from their store in your fat; this must be done with extreme care and sensitivity to what is happening based upon understanding. Do not try to short-circuit the Plan.

Now you have the outline of the Plan, are you ready to take the third step? If you have bathroom scales, throw them away. Remember, we are concerned with the quality of your flesh, not its quantity. Just as your body should not be treated as a rubbish dump, neither should it be thought of as a sack of potatoes. Go back to your mirror, learn to look at yourself, see what you are, recite 'I am the most important thing in my life', and determine to work towards what you want to be.

While carrying out the first two parts of the Plan, detoxification and increasing metabolic capacity, you may not lose any weight at all. On the other hand you might be one of the lucky ones for whom detoxification, or increasing metabolic capacity, is enough in itself to solve the problem. You may even put on a little more weight. Do not panic – this is where you need that cool head! Understand what is going on, and carry on with the Plan.

Whichever way your metabolism reacts, you will start to feel fitter and more energetic with every week you work through. When you do come up to the third part of the Plan, you will find it poses few problems for you – providing you have got the first two stages right.

It is essential that you do not try to go straight to part three. You will not escape. The only route out of PFR is to attend to your toxic intake, then improve the state of your liver. Any other way will just take you back to square one, on the diet/fat see-saw, with more fat than you started. Then you will have to go back to the beginning and start again, because you will have overlooked the fundamental cause for your weight gain. Do it once, and do it right!

If you become ill at any point while working through the Plan, you may have to drop back a stage. Illness puts a demand on the liver; it has to deal with bacteria and the cell and other debris produced when the immune system fights off infections. Put yourself in a holding pattern until the condition has cleared up.

And if you must take medicines, remember they will be putting an additional direct load on your detoxifying systems. See our comments about the advantages and disadvantages of drug usage later.

Illness when you are working on the final phase of the Plan, mobilizing fat, may be an indication that you are pushing yourself too hard. Illness could be your body's way of protesting. Try easing off a little, make progress a little slower. And make absolutely sure you have got the first parts of the Plan covered.

Finally, mobilizing fat and coping with illness, is hard work; make sure you are getting enough good wholesome food to eat, particularly fresh fruit and vegetables. Remember the aim is to work with your body and its systems, not against them.

Detoxification is a gentle process. It means removal from your system and environment of those substances which your metabolism has chosen to treat as toxic. Every individual will react differently to a wide range of potentially toxic substances; you will need to identify those which are causing a problem for you so that you can avoid contact with them. Detailed advice and help with this task is given in chapter 11.

As we have seen, the most important single route for toxic substances into your system is through eating and drinking. Adverse substances in food, drink or medicines can affect you in many ways. Everything we put in our mouths is assessed by our immune systems. If they decide it is safe, no action is taken; if they make a mistake, you may suffer an allergic response; if they decide it is toxic a whole range of defensive mechanisms may swing into action. We are mainly concerned with 'safe' substances that pass through this net.

You will have realized from previous chapters, almost everything you swallow goes through the marshalling yard of the liver for processing. It is here that the crucial overload occurs, and where we must reduce the stress. To do this you will have to be very careful about the substances that you expect your system to process.

The key to success is to realize that things are not always what they seem. If you were asked to judge which was most toxic, a glass of red wine or a glass of malt whisky, the answer might seem simple. Malt whisky has more alcohol, and is therefore more toxic to your system. True – but what if you are sensitive to the sterilizers, inhibitors, colourings or other things which tend to get into some red wines, but will not be found in a good malt?

This is why our dietary advice is based on the idea of innocent food. You should only eat or drink things which have been subject to minimal processing, ideally none at all. Your food should as far as is possible be innocent of any contamination. We will give specific advice on this later. For now let us look at common background problems. Survey after survey has revealed that shoppers judge how fresh and wholesome food is by the packaging. Now while we are sure you are not dumb enough to be taken in by cellophane, bright lights and a slick label, bear in mind that a lot of people are. If they were not, the whole food packaging industry would disappear. The response to this deception is a lucky chance for the food industry. Their main concern is to get products into standard packs, that fit in standard boxes, that load on standard pallets, that fit in standard trucks. It is little wonder that everything possible is done to standardize the food at the beginning of this process. Nature is far from perfect. Reject the packaging, look at what you are going to eat, not at what you are going to throw away.

When did you last see an honest vegetable advertised on the television? As a rough general rule, if they have to advertise foods on television, you should not buy them. To make it all worthwhile such products have to have an entire industry of processing, standardizing, preserving, packaging, warehousing and delivery behind them. Such food is made the way Henry Ford made cars, and you are the scrap heap at the end of the line. Worse, you are expected to pay for the privilege of taking in all the junk!

If you are one of the growing number of people suffering food allergies, the basic contamination of your food may be at the heart of your problem. If you are wrestling with an elimination diet, try our recommendations. It may not be the food after all and your elimination diet could be depriving you of important nutrients. If, however, you confirm that it is the food you are reacting against, then you will have to adapt the dietary rules we give to take account of your particular case. We believe firmly that the foundation of many allergic reactions, from food allergies to hay fever, is the pollution we subject ourselves to, and PFR diet and detoxification strategies will assist with these conditions.

You must also be wary of foods advertised as pure, whole, wholesome, 'with nothing taken out'. This does not mean that nothing has been put in. An increasing number of growers and manufacturers are realizing that there is a growing market for good, wholesome food and drink. Some use every opportunity to bend descriptions as far as they can without breaking the law. Your best guide is to read the labels carefully; your best action is to follow the dietary rules we give in chapter 10.

For most people it remains true that the most potent toxins they are likely to encounter on a day-to-day basis are alcohol and prescribed drugs. Remembering the wine/whisky question, you will have to judge the contribution alcohol might be making to your problem. To assist with prescription drugs, Appendix 2 lists those commonly prescribed drugs acknowledged to cause weight gain in some individuals. However, this list is bound to be incomplete because weight gain may be a side-effect of a particular drug for only a few individuals. The effect may not have been recognized or looked for with other drugs, or it may be an idiosyncratic response.

Drugs are a difficult problem. We are conditioned to believe that they are a universal good and that there is no alternative to their use. If you have to take medication, you may not be able to avoid stressing your liver. You must start by exploring the possibility of not taking the drugs; frequently they are not the best way of dealing with common problems, or even with specific illnesses. There are alternatives to drugs, and we would recommend that you consult a homoeopath for any treatment you may need; the healthy and long-lived Royal family do.

Processing food additives will put a load on your liver. Just look at eleven pounds of flour next time you are in a supermarket and think what the average person in Britain is eating every year in the form of these chemicals. And as this is an average and many people in the know avoid them, try to imagine what quantity some people must consume. Our description of bodies as rubbish dumps is not an exaggeration. We will explain how to cut down on this load, and Appendix 1 has a guide to the hazards of some E-number additives.

The last source of potential toxins we have to deal with is the immediate environment, particularly the air you breathe. We can all control the pollution we release into the air in our homes, and this is the best place to start. You may be naïve enough to believe that there is no pollution in your home – if only that were true!

All those 'cleansers', polishes and sprays and even the 'air fresheners', are nothing short of chemical pollution on the domestic scale. Remember the rule about television advertising, and think what it is that actually makes things shiny, germ-free, 'more fresh, more flowery, smelling more natural than ever before'. That's right, artificial molecules produced by the chemical industry. Their main effects are to fool our senses and confuse our detoxification systems. But you do not have to go along with it. Advice on detoxifying the home without being overrun by germs is given in chapter 11.

If your major problem turns out to be with fumes at work, you may have to consider changing your job. We know this may not be easy, but the choice may be a stark one for you. How much are you willing to suffer and risk for the job and the money it brings? It may be that you can exert pressure to get working conditions improved, but history tends to go against you. It takes an awful lot of dead or deformed before business mends it ways.

Increasing metabolic capacity is not as complicated in practice as it is in theory. You will already have gained some capacity by detoxifying yourself and your immediate environment. The next stage will build on this good work.

If you have been exposed to anything that has damaged your liver, such as a lot of alcohol, you may have a fairly long job on your hands. Fortunately, those highly active and complex liver cells are capable of regeneration under appropriate conditions. And even if you have killed some off, it will be possible to compensate for the losses.

It is crucial to the success of the Plan that you continue to detoxify while you are increasing your metabolic capacity. It is equally important that you do not try to burn any of your toxic adipose tissue off until you have got as much metabolic capacity working for you as you can muster. If you have not got the capacity to cope with the toxins in the adipose tissue, your system will just short-circuit, dumping them straight back into fat.

The lengths you may have to go to to achieve this capacity may seem extreme. Remember you are escaping from a desperate situation. The PFR Syndrome is more common among women because they have livers which are more limited in capacity than those of men. One obvious part of the answer is to redress this imbalance as much as possible.

So it may be necessary to convince your system that you are more masculine than you actually are. By behaving in ways which are subtly more masculine, you will encourage your hormones and liver to respond accordingly. What you will in effect be doing is encouraging your liver to act more like the male liver, building up its capacity to act as a glycogen energy battery. Of course, it will not be able to do this without building up its other capacities – which is the effect we are after.

This will not make you more masculine. Just as your system has been misled by the chemicals which have caused your PFR problem, so the answer may require misleading it a little the other way. You will not get masculine muscles (unless you want them!), nor will you notice any other changes towards maleness.

The principles involved are those which maximize health and healing, and they also bring about improved athletic ability. So even if the idea is a little worrying, the effect will be entirely beneficial. Those who are very overweight may have to spend a little more time and effort on this part of the Plan before finally escaping, but don't worry, you will make it, and stay out permanently.

Mobilizing fat needs care: with PFR your body will not readily let you take off the fat you want to lose. Passive dieting will not work, even starvation will not shift it. You have to burn it off in a controlled manner.

In doing this, you will use your enhanced metabolic capacity. And that hangover effect mentioned earlier will serve as a warning if you attempt to go too fast! It will tell you that you are releasing too much toxic substance into your system. You will have to start off slowly, but as you lose weight, so you will be able to lose it faster.

The only way to mobilize this fat is to burn it up by working your body. This is where your active commitment to losing weight will be really tested. Using your body, being physically active, makes you not only physically competent, but it also enhances the competence of your metabolism. It is in this final phase that you will break through, both to being slim, and to gaining that additional fitness and health which will keep you slim.

Even if you hate the idea, don't despair. Your abhorrence of being physical could be part of a vicious and self-sustaining circle. If you are very overweight, using your body may seem unpleasant, so you will tend to become more overweight. Society's attitudes also militate against you; ladies are supposed to be demure and self-controlled in our culture. But remember, inside you is a vibrant physical animal, capable of pleasure and joy in activity and being. Let yourself go, it is part of your escape from PFR.

Take the opportunity to create the sort of body you have always desired. In chapter 14, after you have solved your PFR problem, we explain the principles behind body shaping, and how you can keep the sort of shape you want for the rest of your life.

That is the outline of the Escape Plan, and we are sure you will agree that it is certainly different. But then so is the problem it is designed to deal with. In the rest of this chapter we will try to anticipate questions that may have come into your mind.

No, the Plan does not involve dieting. By dieting we mean deliberate food restriction which makes you hungry, or sets up cravings for food. This approach to weight loss is counter-productive because it involves fighting your body, making an enemy of it. If dieting were the answer, all those many books, those millions of magazines and the suffering of all those diet addicts, would have produced the slimmest nation in the world; it has not.

We do, however, make specific dietary recommendations. There are certain foods which should be avoided because they are particularly hazardous, either because of the metabolic disruption they induce or because they are likely to be loaded with poisons. Other foods will offer benefits for PFR victims, and details of these are given in chapter 10. But in the end, it is you who has to be in control.

The recommendations we make are aimed at helping you overcome your PFR problem. The Plan offers a balanced diet, a way of eating which anyone susceptible to PFR should try to follow throughout their lives. We believe that it is an eating pattern which will enhance the health and longevity of anyone following it.

How long will it all take? There is no simple answer. Your PFR may have developed over a number of years, perhaps on the diet see-saw, following all those 'quick' diets that took you nowhere; or by the slow accumulation of toxins, after pregnancy or through allergies. If you have been overweight for many years, your bones will have thickened to cope with the additional load, and this will take time to reverse. So it all depends; there are too many individual factors for precise estimates. One thing is sure: the sooner you start, the sooner you will lose that weight.

And it is likely that you will have to accept that without following the Plan you will probably never be able to lose weight fast without making yourself ill. By following it, you will be able to avoid the accumulation of persistent fat in the future, as well as permanently reducing that which you already have.

Because of the permanent nature of the change we are aiming for, you should not rush the Plan. Steady permanent progress, changing to the sort of person you want to be, is the objective. Work on yourself with perseverance and patience. You need to give your body time to readjust its metabolic priorities. A year may seem like an impossibly long time, but is it if at the end of that time you are many pounds lighter, and sure that you need never put that weight on again? How would that compare with what has happened in the year just past? Right, so perhaps spending nine months in preparation, and three months losing pounds is not such a bad outlook.

What about age? It is true that the younger you are, the quicker your healing and regenerative processes tend to be, but this is balanced by the greater tenacity more mature people generally have. People of any age can lose fat – even persistent fat – and help their liver and improve their general health. Too often in our culture we are led to believe that health and vitality are the preserves of the young. Nonsense! What is true is that the older you are, the longer it will tend to take, and the harder you will have to work at it.

We are sure that once you start you will quickly feel much better. You will have more energy and interest in life. Your eyes will be clearer, the whites whiter. And your increasing health will mean that you will want to be more physically active. Once this happens, you will know beyond doubt that you are on the right track. As an added bonus, you will be less likely to suffer those minor infections, and spend less time feeling below par or generally unwell.

CHAPTER 10

The Diet – Innocent Food

What you must eat is food which, beyond any shadow of doubt, is not guilty of causing you any harm. Ideally this means eating organically produced food. This will probably mean making significant changes in your current eating habits and abandoning many of your assumptions about what is good food and what is not. The essential part of the PFR diet is concerned with the quality of what you eat.

The primary aim of the PFR diet is to reduce to the absolute minimum the quantity of artificial chemicals that enter your liver through the digestive system. To do this you have to seek pure, innocent food: food which has been subjected to a minimum of interference during its growth and subsequent processing. Eating such foods will reduce the load on your detoxifying systems, and will also reduce the concentration of chemicals in your blood and tissues.

The second aim of the PFR diet is to provide enough of all the nutrients that you need to rebuild your liver. For this you need adequate quantities of the right foods, and we explain which types are important to you.

Unfortunately, finding pure food is not simple. As we have seen, ordinary food is a chemical minefield. It is one that has to be tackled, however, and success in this area could solve the biggest part of your problem. We believe that most PFR as well as a variety of other metabolic and health problems can be attributed to eating what amounts to poisonous food.

When you follow the PFR diet, you will be cutting your intake of synthetic additives and pesticide residues to the minimum possible. We realize that most people will not be able to live entirely on additive- and residue-free food, and that everyone will want to eat out occasionally, or indulge in their favourite (banned) foods. However, the closer your diet to the ideal described in this chapter, the faster you will achieve detoxification and increased metabolic capacity, and the faster you will be able to lose that persistent fat.

As you grow accustomed to this way of eating, you will find that you prefer it – and you may well wonder how you put up with synthetically flavoured and textureless processed foods for so long. As your body systems improve, you will notice a whole series of benefits accrue from the PFR diet. But that's a general characteristic of all aspects of the Escape Plan!

Avoiding Additives

If you recall the uses to which additives are put, you will already have a very good idea of how to avoid them. The rules are quite simple:

1: Good food is food that will go bad.
You should buy fresh food and eat it at its best. If its best lasts a long time, it is usually because it has been treated with preservatives. The exceptions are dried beans, grains and fruit; these are normally re-hydrated (when they can once more go bad easily) before you actually eat them.

2: The best food is the least processed food.
Obviously, when you pick it off the tree and eat it raw, the processing is minimal. Aim to get food which has had the least done to it. Prepared foods – TV dinners, packet snacks, bakery goods – are usually heavily processed. Fast food does not even

bear thinking about – and you should never, ever, consider eating it.

It is possible to buy prepared foods which are completely free of additives and the range is growing with public demand. Your local wholefood shop is obviously a good source, but more and more high street grocers are stocking up with such foods. Brands to look for include Harmony Foods, Sunwheel, and Höfels, whose tinned vegetable curries and pease pudding can provide instant hot meals.

Read all the small print on labels with great care. Learn the E numbers of the worst additives, or check those on the products you don't want to give up using. One problem area is margarine; many contain additives that could cause you problems.

Another problem is bread. Bread is – or should be – an excellent food, one that we would wholeheartedly recommend. Unfortunately, it is extremely difficult to get additive-free bread in most places. We have tackled this problem by speaking to a small family bakery, promising a firm order of a mutually acceptable number of chemical-free loaves baked from organic flour. Naturally we pay more for these loaves, but believe it's worthwhile.

Your baker may assure you that his stoneground wholemeal bread is fine – but is it? Even if he doesn't add any chemicals, most flour contains preservatives, and the wheat is fumigated with carbon tetrachloride (the liquid used for dry cleaning clothes), a known liver poison which lingers in the flour. If you bake your own, of course, you know what's going into it. Choose your flour carefully and use fresh or dried yeast, not a 'quick' yeast. Another alternative is to buy Springhill organic pumpernickel. It's delicious and sealed into airtight packs which will last.

Cheese is another additive problem area; normally there's no information to guide you, though colours and preservatives are often added. Our advice is that you avoid it or cut your consumption very low. Details on which types to choose if you're a cheese-lover come later in this chapter.

Finally, a word about a substance that you may not think of as a food additive: sugar. Our bodies were never designed to cope with such a substance. Its consumption causes metabolic shock through insulin rebound; one outcome of this is that the body tends to dump sugar molecules into fat – this is why it is known to be fattening. If you want more information on the effects of sugar, read John Yudkin's *Pure, White, and Deadly.* Dark brown sugars and honey are not quite as bad as white sugar, but they can still cause metabolic problems. Avoid them if possible, otherwise restrict your intake to a maximum of two teaspoonsful per day.

Avoiding Pesticide Residues

Ideally, you should only eat organically produced food. That means food that has been grown with organic fertilizers like compost and manure and which has not been treated with synthetic pesticides, and animals that have been reared naturally. This is food produced as an integral part of the biological life-cycle; the waste from natural processes is returned to the soil to enhance its fertility. It is an entirely natural cycle, one that can be sustained without synthetic input indefinitely. It is a method of farming that produces healthy plants and animals and health-enhancing food.

Eating natural, organic food usually means preparing your own food at home. If you habitually eat in restaurants and snack bars, you will have to reorganize your life a little.

We are realists and we know that eating organic food all the time is not possible for most people. Although the network of suppliers is increasing fast, organic food is not available everywhere. You may have to take to buying in bulk on trips to cities, and freezing perishable organic produce when you find it. Your intake of pesticides will be reduced automatically when you follow the PFR diet, but the more of your food that is organically produced, the better.

The first rule of the PFR diet is to avoid all animal fat and internal organs. Like humans, animals store pesticide and drug residues in their fat and organs such as liver, kidneys and heart. Unless you have access to organically reared meat, you should not have more than two meat meals per week, with no more than three ounces of meat at each. Never eat offal. Avoid meat from all animals which have been intensively reared – particularly veal, pork and bacon products and battery chicken. New Zealand lamb is still free-range and has fewer pest problems than British, so this will be less contaminated. Cook it thoroughly to get rid of as much fat as possible, and skim the fat off the cooking juices before making gravy.

Free-range birds and animals are likely to be more free from residues. Wild rabbit, wild duck, venison and, if you are in a country where you can get it, wild boar, can be good food sources. Game from open country should be safe, but avoid pheasants from the over-sprayed lowland grain fields.

You should eat fish about twice weekly. Fish are an excellent form of food because they swim wild and are not dosed with any chemicals – although they can pick them up from the sea through run-off from fields and chemical pollution from industry. Avoid farmed fish such as trout; go for cod, haddock, sole, herring, skate, monkfish, dogfish and catfish. Mackerel is not recommended because it has relatively high residue levels. Buy from a good fishmonger, not in cans or frozen, and never eat fish fingers. Avoid 'smoked' fish, which is usually coloured with coal-tar dye. Never take fish liver oil dietary supplements: fish livers are highly polluted. If you are eating out, fish can be a good choice.

Most dairy produce is polluted with residues, but you can avoid the worst of them by choosing only low-fat forms. Do not eat butter and substitute good quality cold-pressed oils such as olive and sunflower for cooking. Choose skimmed milk, low-fat natural yoghurt, and low-fat cheeses such as Edam, Gouda and Camembert. Avoid cottage cheese, even if it is low-fat, unless you are sure it does not contain preservatives; the leading brands do. Use goat or sheep milk products whenever possible;

these are often available from delicatessens and Greek shops as well as from health food stores. If you hate goat's milk, do try sheep's – they taste quite different.

Eggs are included in the PFR diet because they contain vitamins and amino acids that are essential to good liver function. But you must buy free-range. You will get a less polluted egg, and the vitamin levels are much higher. The flavour's incomparably better too! We recommend that you eat between three and seven eggs a week, boiled or poached, but do not fry them.

Proteins are important to good liver function and the least polluted sources are vegetable. Remember that whole grains, nuts, seeds, peas and beans provide good sources of protein, but you can be sure of an unpolluted source of essential health-other grains with peas, beans or nuts to get the right balance.

Nuts and seeds (particularly sunflower seeds) are very good in salads, or for nibbling. They play an important part in the PFR diet, as we'll explain later.

Fresh vegetables complement vegetable protein foods and together these form the core of the PFR diet. You should aim to eat a salad every day because cooking removes valuable nutrients from many vegetables; your salads should contain a handful of sprouted beans, grains or seeds as well as the more familiar leaves, roots and vegetable fruits. You will be sprouting these yourself, in the kitchen or airing cupboard, because that way you can be sure of an unpolluted source of essential health-giving nutrients every day.

For those who have not tried sprouting, here's how you start. Buy some mung beans from your local good food shop. Put a tablespoon of them in a wide-mouthed jar. Cover them with plenty of boiled water, cooled down to blood heat. Put the jar in a warm dark place. After twenty-four hours, pour off the water and rinse your beans thoroughly. Then, every twelve hours or so, rinse the sprouting beans under the tap, draining off all the water you can and returning them to the jar. After three days or so, your beans will have sprouts about an inch and a half long, and fresh green leaves just showing. Put the jar on your window sill for a day. Now your sprouts are ready to eat – preferably raw, but lightly stir-fried if you must cook them. You will find that the tablespoon of beans you started with has produced two handfuls of sprouts – enough for you for two days! It's the cheapest form of food we know, as well as one of the most nutritious.

The same basic method can be used for grains such as wheat and rye, for sunflower seeds, and for other types of beans. More details are given in Leslie and Susannah Kenton's excellent books, *Raw Energy* and *Raw Energy Recipes*. They are well worth buying for their original salad ideas alone – and will prove very useful to you when you're applying the rules of the PFR diet to your life.

Most of your food – including the beans and seeds you'll need for sprouting – will come from your local wholefood or health food shop. But be wary, they can also carry esoteric junk in the name of health, or imports of dubious origin. Study the label, or question the staff carefully, to ensure that you are getting unsprayed, organically grown food whenever possible, because there are still comparatively few shops that sell only organic.

Some grocers and supermarkets (notably Safeway) are beginning to stock organic and wholefood lines. Encourage them by asking for things they do not yet have on the shelves. Again read labels carefully. And avoid those supermarkets that find it necessary to pollute their entire premises with chemical cleaners in the name of hygiene. It is totally unnecessary and only adds to your problem. (We watched the inside of a fully stocked cheese cabinet being sprayed with 'cleanser'! Not a very fine way to treat fare.)

Your best guarantees of pure food are the symbols shown below. These approval marks are only awarded to growers whose methods, produce and soil meet very stringent standards. Also any food which is marked 'bio-dynamic' should be pesticide-free and highly nutritious. But beware of Eddie Grundy-type opportunists!

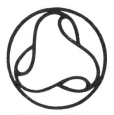

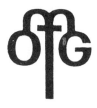

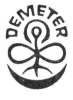

Soil Association
Symbol of Organic Quality

Organic Farmers
and Growers

Bio-Dynamically
grown organic
food

Fresh produce may not have these guarantees and you will have to rely on the integrity of the shop or market trader. If it is sold as 'organic', it should contain no pesticide residues. But remember, 'wholefoods' and 'health foods' are no more likely to be pesticide-free than any others unless they are specifically marked as such.

Strangely enough, your best guarantee may be things which are usually thought of as pests. If there are greenflies on the lettuce, the odd caterpillar in the cabbage, or even a maggot in an apple, you can be fairly sure that, if it is safe for them, it is safe for you. Try looking upon these humble creatures as the modern equivalent of the miner's canary. While the canary sang down the pit, the men knew they were safe from poisonous gas. Where insects are happy, you are safe; where they are being poisoned, so are you.

Luckily, there are certain old-established brands whose food has managed to retain its integrity. Again, their products may not always be 100 per cent organic, but the label will state this where it is the case. You should make a note of the names, and ask for their produce as often as possible, and buy them as a matter of course.

Look for Pimhill, Hofels Pure Foods, Infinity Foods, Sunwheel Foods, Harmony Foods and Johanus products. Organic flours are available from various millers; we recommend Dove's Farm wholewheat flour – it makes the most delicious bread. If you have difficulty in finding stockists, the addresses of these firms are in Appendix 3 (a stamped addressed envelope with your inquiry would probably be appreciated).

If you can get to London, there are two notable centres of organic food you should patronize. One is the Neal's Yard complex in Covent Garden – a greengrocer, a bakery, a dairy, a grocery, a herbalist, and a French food shop. The other is Wholefood of Paddington Street, a shop founded by members of The Soil Association. Here you will find everything from this book and many others, to all the organic produce you could want, including a supply of fresh fruit and vegetables. You will also find the staff enthusiastic, knowledgeable and helpful. There is an organic butcher's shop a few doors down from the main store. If you want uncontaminated meat, from animals which were not abused when alive, this is your shop. We can recommend the liver!

More organic suppliers are springing up all the time, so do not assume you cannot get organic food just because we have not included a shop in your town in the list. Further information is available in *The Organic Food Guide*, edited by Alan Gear.

While things are getting better, it will be true that most of us will not be able to obtain enough organic food to meet all our needs. So here are some tips which may help. Have you seriously thought about growing more of your own food? Any garden can support salad crops and you get them totally fresh and crisp. Lettuces and radishes are the easiest to grow, and fruits such as strawberries need very little attention. You can also eat any part of the nasturtium plant – use the leaves and flowers in salads and pickle the seeds to eat with your fish.

The important thing to remember is that you must maintain a very high level of organic material in the soil, especially if you live in a town. If you do not, you will not be able to produce nourishing crops. If you are anywhere near a road and there is not enough organic material in the soil, your crops could contain lead from car exhausts. Start a compost heap, collect leaf-mould, dig in manure to build high levels of fertility. Many books are available on the subject; we rely on Laurence Hills' *Organic Gardening*.

If you can get an allotment, you can grow enough fresh food to feed a family for most of the year. This may mean that you spend some Sunday hours, as we do, working the soil; but it is a very relaxing and uniquely satisfying way of spending time. And use hand tools, do not join the feeble motor-on-everything brigade who pollute with fumes and noise. You will be a lot fitter and slimmer!

If you don't fancy gardening, and there isn't a good food shop near you, why not think about opening one? Many of the big alternative food distribution coops and stores started just like this. Try an advertisement in the local press to find like-minded entrepreneurs.

If none of these suggestions are feasible, you will need to protect yourself as best you can by choosing food that is least likely to be polluted with pesticides. Here are some guidelines:

Avoid frozen and tinned food wherever possible. The manufacturers of these products demand produce that looks absolutely perfect, and the farmers therefore spray more thoroughly.

Always peel or thoroughly scrape potatoes; they are not only sprayed repeatedly during growing, but usually treated after harvesting with chemicals that prevent sprouting.

Buy 'new' potatoes, carrots and other vegetables when you have a choice. Select early crops rather than stored produce. For example, when you have a choice of new-crop Spanish onions or stored English onions in the summer, buy Spanish: they are less likely to have been sprayed with growth inhibitors.

Never buy brightly-coloured dried fruit; the colour is the product of preservatives. Choose brownish apricots – especially the delicious little Hunzas, and sun-dried, oil-free raisins.

British may not be best for minimizing residues. If you have a choice, buy product from France, Holland, Scandinavia or

New Zealand, where farmers' spraying behaviour tends to be more moderate. It may be wise to avoid Italian and Mexican produce.

Now you know how to avoid the chemicals that will tend to put a load on your liver, you will need to know about the other side of the diet: the specific nutrients that will help your escape from the PFR Syndrome.

The nutrients described here are essential to the Plan. You must not skimp on the foods which contain them. While you do not have to eat all the foods in each group (Tables 1 to 4), you should make sure you do have some of them every day.

Do not imagine you can get away with taking supplements instead; your body may not respond to a synthetic nutrient and could even treat it as yet another toxic additive in your diet!

Liver – as you might guess – is a rich source of many of the nutrients you will need. Unfortunately, it is also a concentrated source of all the poisons to which the animal has been exposed. If you can get naturally reared, organic liver, it will be beneficial; but the product from the local butcher or supermarket is more likely to be harmful.

Iron is crucial for effective de-toxification. It is used in one of the liver's metabolic cycles. Sources are given in Table 1. If you avoid drinking tea, coffee or soft drinks with your meals, this will increase the amount of iron your body can take up from your food. Avoiding food additives also improves your iron uptake, so if you have tended to be anaemic in the past, the PFR diet should remedy the problem.

Folic acid, one of the B group vitamins, is essential for building new liver tissue and replacing cells throughout the body. Sources are in Table 2.

Vitamin C is necessary for healing. Table 3 lists good sources. Unfortunately, vitamin C disappears from foods with storage, and the quantity available from most sources falls in winter. This is when you will be relying on bean and grain sprouts – you should eat more in the winter months. Sprouts also contain other vitamins and trace minerals which will help your escape from PFR: the sprouting process increases the quantity available many-fold.

The amino acids cysteine and methionine are absolutely essential to your success. Cysteine is denatured by cooking, so you must incorporate some raw sources into your diet every day. Brazil nuts are exceptionally rich in both these amino acids, but you must be sure they are fresh. Other sources are given in Table 4.

Table 1: Foods rich in iron

Vegetable sources

butter beans	haricot beans	mung beans
lentils	peas	broccoli
leeks	radishes	spring greens
watercress	parsley	

Fruit sources

dried apricots	dried figs	prunes
blackcurrants	redcurrants	raspberries
loganberries	raisins	

Nuts (except chestnuts); dark-coloured meat

Table 2: Foods rich in folic acid

Vegetable sources

cabbage, broccoli, brussels sprouts and other brassicas (raw)

beetroot	endive	chicory
lettuce	spring onions	spinach
sweetcorn	watercress	

Fruit sources

avocado pears	melons (all types)	oranges

Other good sources

free-range eggs	almonds	walnuts

Table 3: Foods rich in vitamin C

Vegetable sources

potatoes – the newer the better

asparagus	beansprouts	broccoli
brussels sprouts	cabbage	cauliflower
kale	mustard and cress	radishes
watercress	mint	parsley

Fruit sources

blackcurrants	gooseberries	melon

citrus fruit (oranges, grapefruit, lemons, satsumas, etc.)

lychees	mangoes	guavas

fresh pineapple

all berry fruits (raspberries, strawberries, blackberries, etc.)

Table 4: Foods rich in cysteine and/or methionine

eggs	brazil nuts	sunflower seeds
cashew nuts	walnuts	sweetcorn
millet	rice	wheat
fish		

Applying the principles of the PFR diet

These are the rules you must follow:

1. Forget everything you have ever thought about dieting.
It is almost certain to be just the sort of psychological baggage that will hinder your escape from the PFR Syndrome. Leave it behind.

2. You must be absolutely sure that you eat enough food.
Your body has a lot of work to do, both in detoxifying and in rebuilding your liver. It will not be able to do it if you keep it short of fuel. Eat plenty of the foods in the tables above!

3. Forget about your weight – look at your shape.
You may find that the quantities of food we recommend are greater than you have been in the habit of eating, and you may fear putting on weight. This is a possibility in the short term,

while you are rebuilding your liver. Accept this without worrying. You will find that a higher level of metabolic health will mean that you have more energy and you will start to burn more food. If you have been in the habit of restricting your food intake, your metabolic rate will be depressed. Eat more of the right foods, follow the Plan, and it will increase.

The PFR Escape Plan calls for two different meal schedules. Schedule 1 is the one you'll start with, and you may need to stay with this indefinitely. Certainly, you should keep to Schedule 1 for the first two stages of the Plan (detoxification and mobilizing your metabolism). It requires that you eat many small meals each day and nibble whenever you're peckish. Forget about avoiding between-meal snacks; have as many as you want. But always choose the foods that are recommended in the tables.

Schedule 2 is for those who have rebuilt their liver and are ready to increase its capacity. It is to be used with the activity regime described in the final stages of the Plan. It is designed to run down your liver glycogen stores and build them up again on a cyclical basis, so it calls for just one main meal a day and periods of fasting or very light eating at other times. It is not likely to suit you if you have passed middle age; older people should not cut down to fewer than three meals a day.

Our week-by-week action plan (chapter 13) will explain precisely when you should consider changing from Schedule 1 to Schedule 2. Both schedules demand that you eat the same basic foods, but the balance is changed as you progress. So the first thing you need to know is what foods to eat, and in what quantities.

We cannot give strict rules on quantities. As we have already emphasized, there is tremendous individual variability in food needs, and you will have to judge for yourself when you have had enough. Just remember the second rule: always eat enough food! This is easier when you follow the PFR diet because you will not be confusing your body with processed foods which don't provide the signals that tell you when you've had what you need.

We have divided the foods into YES, PERHAPS and NO. You will be relying on the YES group throughout; PERHAPS foods are to be eaten with caution; they are not essential, and you should not have large quantities. You should try to avoid NO foods completely; they are likely to contain chemicals which will interfere with your progress.

These lists are not comprehensive – we could not make them so. They are intended for guidance and you will have to work out which group other foodstuffs would fall into by reference to the lists and the text above.

Table 5: YES Foods

These are your staple foods and they should be eaten every day. If you are allergic to any particular types, substitute others from the same group.

Food type	Varieties	Cooking method	Quantity	Comments
sprouts	bean, seed or grain	raw or stir-fried	1 handful	home-grown
green salad	any fresh vegetables, home-grown if possible	raw	as much as you like	watercress recommended
brassicas	broccoli, cauliflower, cabbage, brussels, kale	raw or steamed	as much as you like	
roots	potatoes	boiled or baked	8–14oz	new if available
	carrots, beet, swede, turnip, etc.	raw or boiled	as much as you like	
legumes	fresh peas or beans	lightly boiled	as much as you like	
	butter beans, lentils, haricot beans, red beans	boiled or in soups	1 cup cooked	soak and boil hard
other vegetables	leeks, onions, etc.	as desired	as desired	

MISCELLANEOUS PROTEIN SOURCES

seeds	sunflower, pumpkin	raw or sprouted	2oz daily	nibble; good in salads
nuts	cashews, brazils, walnuts	raw	2oz	
eggs	free-range	not fried	max. 1 daily	
yoghurt	natural, goat or sheep milk		5oz	
fish	fresh, not smoked	any	4–8oz	

FRUIT

	any fresh fruit	raw	½ to 1lb	soft fruit recommended; avoid citrus peel
dried fruit	Hunza apricots other unsulphured fruit	raw or boiled	1–2oz	delicious with yoghurt

GRAINS

	rolled oats	muesli or porridge	1–2oz	
	wheat/rye	bread pasta	2–4 slices as desired	wholegrain
	brown rice	boiled	as desired	

OIL

	olive or sunflower	for cooking and salads	as required	cold-pressed

SEASONINGS

salt	sea salt	use sparingly	
	pepper, spices herbs	as desired	
	tahini tamari soy sauce	as desired as desired	
	lemon juice, cider vinegar	as desired	avoid preservatives

Table 6: PERHAPS Foods

Food type	Varieties	Cooking method	Quantity	Comments
milk cheese	skimmed milk, goats' milk low fat cheeses	as required	max. ½ pint max. 2oz	choose goats' or sheep's
meat	poultry or game lamb lambs' liver	as desired remove fat grilled or casseroled	3oz 3oz weekly 3oz	free-range New Zealand organic only
breakfast cereals	Weetabix, Grapenuts, Shredded Wheat, Puffed Wheat, other sugar-free cereals		normal helping	organic oats preferable

Table 7: NO Foods

Avoid these as far as possible – although if you find organic or additive-free varieties, they will be fine.

Food	Varieties	Comments
dairy produce	full cream cow's milk cream, full fat cheeses	residues in fat
	fruit/nut yoghurt ice cream	contains sugar, additives contains sugar, additives
meat	beef, pork, veal, chicken, turkey, etc	residues in fat
breakfast cereals	sweetened forms, corn flakes, bran cereals, etc.	contain sugar, additives
flour products	Biscuits, cakes, puddings white bread	contain sugar, additives contains bleach, additives
desserts, sweets, confectionery, jams	shop-bought types	contain sugar, additives except Whole Earth jams – but still max. 1 teaspoon
Sauces and dressings (including those integrated in foods, e.g. baked beans, pasta, etc.)	shop-bought types	except Whole Earth or additive- and sugar-free forms

Creating Menus

Schedule 1

The menus suggested below are, once again, for guidance. You do not need to stick to them if you can think of ways you'd prefer to make your YES foods into day-to-day meals.

On rising
Herb tea, bottled spring water, or 50:50 water and fruit juice

Breakfast
½ grapefruit (no sugar)
Bowl of organic porridge (no milk or sugar). We make porridge for two with 1 cup organic breakfast oats, 2½ cups water, ½ teaspoon sea salt, 1 dessertspoon organic oat or wheat bran. It's delicious on its own – nothing needs to be added!

or
Small bowl organic muesli with skimmed milk or yoghurt

or
Stewed Hunza apricots with organic wheatgerm and yoghurt

or
Boiled or poached egg with wholemeal toast

Elevenses
1 slice wholemeal bread with margarine, olive oil or tahini

or
Sunflower seeds and fresh fruit

or
Natural yoghurt

Lunch
Sprouted seed and fresh vegetable salad with wholemeal bread or pumpernickel

or
Split pea or lentil soup with wholemeal croûtons

or
Brown rice with stir-fried vegetables

Tea
Fresh fruit and nuts or seeds

or
Pumpernickel with raw sprouts

Dinner
Baked or grilled with vegetables

or
Boiled egg with potatoes and salad

or
Free-range poultry with baked potato and vegetables or salad

or
Chilli beans with rice and salad

or
Organic wholewheat pasta with tahini and vegetable sauce, seafood sauce or tomato sauce with 1oz finely grated Gouda cheese

or
Cabbage leaves, pepper, aubergine, or young marrow stuffed with rice, nuts, tomatoes and shallots (Greek recipes are very good – but halve the quantity of oil!)

or
Bean and vegetable stew

Fresh fruit

General comments
You should make sure you have at least one helping of fresh salad every day. In winter, your bean, grain and seed sprouts will dominate your salads, but many winter vegetables such as roots can be grated and added to your salads. If you're starting to grow a little food in your garden, include American cress and lambs' lettuce for winter greenstuff.

Vary your salads with vegetables you normally cook – such as grated young swedes and turnips (delicious with chopped apricots and walnuts) or raw courgettes, flowers such as marigolds and nasturtiums from the garden. Make dressings with natural yoghurt and herbs, cold-pressed oil and lemon juice (watch for preservatives), liquidized avocado and wine vinegar. *Raw Energy* (see Recommended Books, p. 184) has many imaginative suggestions.

Try going Chinese: stir-fry cashew nuts with finely chopped vegetables in a little oil; season with Tamari or other naturally fermented soy sauce. Other cultures – both Eastern and Near Eastern – have traditions of eating in ways that will fit in well with your PFR diet.

Potential problems
You're desperate for a biscuit, but you know they're forbidden. Have an oatcake; buy a sugar-free brand such as Patterson's.

You passionately want something sweet – like chocolate. Try carob-coated raisins (not too many) or chew a couple of dried figs. Avoid the sweetened supermarket version – we can't imagine how anyone would want to make figs even sweeter than they are!

You long for your favourite junk snack. This can be more difficult because you may be addicted to the additives and sugar in processed foods. They give your body a jolt that can be experienced as a 'high' related to that you might get with certain drugs. The mechanism is similar; these substances pervert your metabolic processes for their own end, and just as withdrawal from drugs can be difficult, so can withdrawal from processed foods for those who have become dependent on them. Recognize your addition for what it is – and acknowledge that it could be the major cause of your PFR problem. Do not give in: search determinedly for additive-free substitutes and don't allow yourself to go hungry. Hunger could help your will-power to be undermined.

Gradually remove all temptation of this sort from your house; wean your family off it, they will benefit too. After a while, you will find such foods taste just as revolting as they are. Nobody will be able to fob you off with any synthetic imitations of real, flavoursome food any more!

Schedule 2

By the time you get this far, you will be totally accustomed to eating on the PFR diet. The changes you will be making now are not fundamental; it's a question of changing the balance of your diet.

On Schedule 2, you will be very physically active, and you will want to eat more food. Do not increase your consumption of protein foods such as fish, eggs and nuts; choose more complex carbohydrates – particularly grains and root vegetables.

Breakfast
Piece of fruit
Small bowl porridge or muesli

Elevenses
1 cup coffee if desired

Lunch
As Schedule 1

Tea
2 slices wholemeal bread with fresh sprouts or salad vegetables
Piece of fresh fruit
Sunflower seeds or nuts

Dinner
Lentil, split pea or vegetable soup
or
Melon, grapefruit or avocado

Main course as Schedule 1, but double portions of potato, rice, pasta, bean and vegetable stew

Fresh and/or dried stewed fruit, or baked apple stuffed with dried fruit and 1 teaspoon of honey, with yoghurt.
or
Fruit pie or additive-free pudding (sweetened with concentrated apple juice or dried fruit)

Oatcakes, pumpernickel or bread with 1oz low-fat cheese if desired

Drink
Now you have the rules for eating, you will be wondering what to wash it down with. There's no point in detoxifying one part of your intake and ruining the effect by pouring in liquid hazards!

The most important rule is that you drink enough water. Drink just as much of this as you like, at any time of the day. Never restrict your liquid intake: this will interfere with detoxification.

Sensible people stick to those drinks that will help their systems rather than add to the load on them. Pure spring water sold in glass bottles is good for your liver and digestion, and delicious too.

Fresh fruit and vegetable juices (not squashes) are also

excellent. But read the labels – junk abounds in drinks. Go for purity. Citrus juices contain valuable vitamin C, necessary for healing and detoxification, and carrot juice is rich in vitamin A. It is possible to get organic fruit juice; check the labels on bottles in your local wholefood store and stock up with the types you prefer. Holle and Johanus juices are uncontaminated, but these are not the only brands you may find. Dilute juices 50:50 with water.

Coffee, tea and chocolate may cause you problems and can interfere with your efforts to detoxify your body and improve liver function. You would be wise to give up drinking them and substitute herb teas. Lime flower, camomile, marigold and mint teas may be particularly helpful. When you reach Schedule 2, you may be able to drink one or two cups of tea and/or coffee a day without harming your progress, but don't let the quantities build up.

Hazards: soft drinks – low calorie or otherwise – are completely banned. PFR victims may be particularly vulnerable to such products. These concoctions of colours, flavourings and sweeteners merely add to your chemical load. The same goes for milk shakes. Don't touch them!

Milk, and dairy products generally, should be used only minimally. Contaminated animal fats are concentrated in most dairy products. Strawberries, yes, cream – no! And don't replace milk with non-dairy creamer – it's a totally unnatural chemical product. Avoid drinking tea and coffee, and you'll rarely want milk. What milk you do use should be skimmed, or goat's.

Tap water is going downhill. It is assumed to be safe, but, as the prevarication by the Water Authorities faced with new EEC regulations demonstrates, it can be hazardous. Ours is too hard to pass through kidneys without complaint. It might be advisable to filter your water before use. Water filter jugs and constant flow filters are readily available; they make your water a refreshing drink once more.

You will realize that alcohol is likely to pose particular

problems for PFR sufferers. Obviously, your best option is to avoid all alcohol. Some will already have made this decision, having observed that alcohol makes them unwell. Others will reject this option as unrealistic and unacceptable. If you will not abstain from alcohol, then the next best option is to choose the least hazardous forms, drink only occasionally and then in moderation. Go for quality and flavour.

Rapidly-produced, cheap forms of alcoholic drink will contain not only alcohols of various types, but a whole range of other substances such as sulphites. Large-scale brewing and wine-making is now a chemically controlled process, and residues remain in the end product.

Good quality wines, and especially the French 'biologique' wines, produced without the use of chemicals in growing or fermentation, are likely to cause your body fewer problems than poorer ones. White, in general, is more easily metabolized than red wine. If you have noticed that you tend to get a particularly nasty hangover after certain drinks, avoid those completely.

Good quality spirits are often purer than longer drinks. We prefer single malt whiskies from Scotland's smaller distilleries. These are still made in the traditional manner, to give a pure flavour reminiscent of the lovely, if bracing, windswept moors where they originated.

If you do have a few drinks at a celebration, you should help your liver to cope with the load as quickly and efficiently as possible. Take plenty of water or pure fruit juice between alcoholic drinks, and dance energetically for at least twenty minutes to burn up the alcohol. Perhaps a brisk walk home, instead of the car, could have the same effect. The worst thing to do is to sit or stand about drinking, cocktail-party style, and then go to bed. Your efforts to improve liver function will receive a severe setback every time you allow this to happen.

Finally, if you are offered a slice of lemon with your drink, refuse it. The peel will almost certainly be polluted with fungicides that will dissolve in your drink. Some of those sprayed on citrus fruits are the most hazardous in common use.

As for 'cocktail cherries' . . . You just have to look at the colour of those things to know they won't do you any good at all. No thanks!

CHAPTER 11

Detoxification

Few people think about the way the everyday chemicals they encounter may affect them. But toxins reach your liver and your fat stores through a variety of other routes besides the food and drink you consume. They will add to your personal loading and exacerbate the problem.

In addition to food additives, drugs and pesticides, the chemical industry produces a vast range of substances which end up in your environment. These range from household cleansers, polishes and sprays, to personal products such as deodorizers and perfumes, as well as a wide range of office and industrial products. For PFR victims it is ironic that they may be persuaded to buy things to pollute their environment by being led to believe that such products are highly desirable, if not indispensable.

For some people environmental toxins may be more critical than those in food and drink we have emphasized previously. The only way to be sure is to minimize your exposure to both.

Because of our individual differences in metabolism, it is not possible to predict the most important sources for everybody; you will be relatively more sensitive to one group of chemicals, less affected by another. With your growing knowledge of yourself and your growing understanding of the nature of the problem, you may begin to identify particular groups which adversely affect you.

In this chapter, we explain how and where you can identify

some of the most common sources of environmental toxins. The first part concerns your home – and we predict that you will be shocked to discover just how many toxic threats it contains! Do the questionnaire below to find out.

Arm yourself with a notepad and pen, put on some old clothes and set off on the hunt. (Kids and other members of the household can join in, it could be made into a good rainy afternoon game!)

1. Count all the aerosol sprays in your home.
  a. Check your personal items – hair sprays, deodorants, medicines, shaving cream, etc. How many aerosol cans are there? ....
  b. Now check fabric care sprays such as starch, dry-cleaning and proofing products. How many of these? ....
  c. How many spray polishes and cleaners? ....
  d. How many spray paints, varnishes, and dyes? ....
  e. How many cans of air freshener or room deodorizer? ....
  f. How many cans of fly spray, pet flea spray, household insecticide spray? ....
  g. Do you use any other sprays in the kitchen, e.g. coatings for cooking vessels? How many of these? ....

2. Do you use washing powder that contains enzymes (that means almost all types except pure soap or Original Non-biological Persil)?

3. Do you use products which leave your clothes perfumed (including fabric conditioners)?

4a. Do you regularly wear dry-cleaned clothes?
  b. Does your partner wear dry-cleaned clothes?
  c. Are any of your furnishings dry-cleaned?

5. Do you use long-lasting or block deodorizers (e.g. in the lavatory or kitchen)? Check your lavatory paper – we

recently bought, in error, some perfumed rolls which made us sneeze!

6. Do you use long-lasting insecticides?

7. Do you use insecticidal pet shampoo, or does your pet wear a flea collar?

8. Do you use strong-smelling glues (such as Evostick) in the house?

9. Is there any new paint in the house (painted within six weeks)?

10. Do you have urea-formaldehyde cavity foam insulation in the walls of your home?

11. Has the timber in your home been treated with preservative within the past year?

12. Do you have plastic-covered furniture?

13. Do you have flexible plastic clothing, shower curtains, tablecloths, etc?

Now check the places you regularly go outside: the garage, garden shed, and car.

14. Do you have a new car?

15. Do you use cellulose paints?

16. Do you use paint or varnish strippers?

17. Is there an air freshener in your car?

18. Do you use pesticides in the garden?

Finally, back in the house, check your heating and cooking facilities.

19. Do you have gas heaters or a gas cooker?

20. Do you use paraffin or bottled gas heaters?

Now check your chemical contaminant rating:

Question 1: All aerosol sprays are capable of causing problems. Count 1 for each can you find.
Question 2: Add 5 for biological washing powder.
Question 3: Occasional use, add 2; regular use, add 5.
Question 4a: Add 2 for each day of past fortnight when you wore clothes dry-cleaned within a month.
4b: Add 1 for each day your partner wore recently dry-cleaned clothes in past fortnight.
4c: Add 2 per item of furniture, carpets, curtains, dry-cleaned within the past 6 months.
Question 5: Add 2 per item.
Question 6: Add 5 per item.
Question 7: Add 2 per flea collar; 2 per use of shampoo within the past 6 weeks.
Question 8: Add 4 for each use within the past 6 weeks.
Question 9: Add 4 for each room repainted within the past 6 weeks; plus 4 if you did the painting.
Question 10: Add 10 if yes.
Question 11: Add 20 if yes.
Question 12: Add 10 for furniture less than 1 year old; 2 per item more than 1 year old. (Count only flexible coverings.)
Question 13: Add 4 per item less than 1 year old; 2 per item over 1 year old.
Question 14: Add 4 for a car less than 1 year old.
Question 15: Add 6 for each use within the past 6 weeks.

Question 16: Add 6 for each use within the past 6 weeks.
Question 17: Add 2 if yes.
Question 18: Add 2 for each type.
Question 19: Add 20 if you can smell gas anywhere in the house. And whether or not you can smell gas, add 2 for every gas heating or cooking appliance.
Question 20: Add 2 for every bottled gas or paraffin heater.

Now check your rating.

Over 140
Your home is heavily contaminated with chemicals. Check which sources are most significant and start working immediately on eliminating them. Specific advice comes later in this chapter.

You are overanxious about dirt, pests, and natural smells. Perhaps you take undue notice of the heavy advertising that is designed to make you buy, buy, buy? Remember that a chemical, 'fresh' smell is likely to be damaging to your health and figure and use your nose to judge the hazard. Anything you can smell is present in the air you breathe, and it goes straight into your bloodstream from the membranes of your nose and lungs.

A chemically-coated surface may be germ-free and it may look good – but that doesn't make it clean or healthy.

If you've been doing a lot of painting and house renovation, you will have been exposed to a heavy chemical load and you may not be willing to stop the work yet. Protect yourself by keeping the house, car, garage or shed very well ventilated. Leave all the doors and windows open as much as you can, let fresh air waft the poisons away.

90 to 140
The chemical contamination level of your home is high and is likely to cause you problems if you are at all susceptible. Probably you have a heavy loading from some sources and little problem with others. Think about why you use so many

chemicals: is it convenience, ignorance of their dangers, an over-conscientious attitude to cleaning and polishing?

Now you've been alerted to the major sources of chemical contaminants in your home environment, you will be more aware of them. Throw away as many as you can, stop using others, go back to methods that your grandmother might have used.

40 to 90

You are not an excessive user of chemicals, but you still have more sources of contamination in your home than you really need. Whether they prove a problem to you depends on your personal sensitivity; you might be reacting very badly to particular sources so that the limited range in your home still represents too much for your detoxifying systems.

Focus on any products that make you sneeze or feel in any way unwell, and get rid of them. Then gradually reduce your use of other potential sources of problems.

Under 40

The level of contamination in your home is well below average, and it may not represent a problem for you unless you are sensitive to particular sources.

If, however, you suffer from any allergies, especially hay fever or asthma, you will need to look critically at every single item that contaminates the air you breathe. The chances are that you can live without them.

Everybody who suffers from persistent fat or any allergic problems should do their very best to reduce their household pollution score to 20 or less.

Here are some tips:

Washing and cleaning

A generation ago, most of the cleaning products we use now had not been invented. They come from the enormous petro-chemical industry, where new compounds are developed all the time and sold to the public with clever marketing that is designed to exploit our fears of 'dirt' or 'germs' and social unacceptability.

For many people, probably including you, the contamination they substitute in return for removing these hazards has a far worse effect than the original problem. They are sold by appealing to implied social values; so you may have to shake out some more unwanted psychological baggage.

Does a pair of grass-stained shorts on your child really make you into a slut, as the detergent advertisements imply? Surely your first priority is to keep your children fit and well – not glazed and gleaming. Bright, white washing comes second after health. Be clean without being obsessive. And if the main purpose in your life is a washing-line competition with your neighbour, aren't both of you wasting your lives?

Never have anything dry-cleaned if you can wash it. Often you can ignore labels on clothing that say 'dry-clean only'. In our experience, hand washing with a gentle liquid product or pure soap rarely does any damage; most warnings are quite unnecessary. Test a small part where it won't matter if the colour runs to see if it can actually stand washing.

If clothes really must be dry-cleaned, hang them outside to air for as long as possible before you put them away or wear them. And when you're choosing clothes or furnishings, pick those that can be washed. Nobody needs to be exposed to poisonous fumes from dry-cleaning solvents.

Dry-cleaning fluids – including those you use at home – are known to cause liver problems. Sensitive people have been shown to have high levels of these chemicals in their blood after wearing or being close to dry-cleaned clothes or furnishings.

On cleaning generally:

For you the answer to smells and odours is not in bottles or sprays. Use old fashioned soap and water, re-discover washing soda, use natural perfumes wherever you can. Cut out everything else ruthlessly. If you have body odour problems, you will find as you become healthier and less contaminated you will naturally leave much of this problem behind. It may be caused by the chemicals you are using to solve it!

For your home, a damp cloth and vacuum cleaner will cope with almost everything.

When replacing clothes, fabrics and furnishings, go for things which do not require complicated cleaning and care routines.

One final word on cleaning: rinse everything thoroughly. Never add anything to the final rinsing water (except natural products such as lemon juice or vinegar for brightness). And that applies to you as well as your washing-up or clothes. You will not benefit from having any part of yourself or your environment covered with a chemical film – even if it does give a nice shine.

A general avoidance of all perfumes except those from known natural sources is wise. Avoid synthetically perfumed cosmetics, soaps, cleaning products; instead, make your house smell sweet with plants, rose petals and herbs such as lavender. Handle cut flowers – especially long-lasting ones like chrysanthemums – with care; some have such high levels of pesticide on them that they have poisoned florists!

Plastic fabrics and fabric coatings are hazardous because the chemicals used to make them flexible slowly evaporate into the air. When they've finally gone and the product is safe, it's stiff and liable to tear – which is when we throw it away.

One of the most potentially dangerous plastics is PVC. The chemical which leaches out of it is vinyl chloride, which is known to cause cancer and liver disease. PVC is used in flexible food containers and many other items such as plastic baby pants. The safest option is to avoid everything made of flexible plastic.

The familiar smell of a new car is the smell of plasticizers which evaporate from seat coverings and other interior furnishings. If you buy a new car, leave all the doors open as often as possible, especially in warm weather. Drive with the windows open until the smell disappears.

Plastics come in a great many different forms. We cannot hope to give an exhaustive list here. Let your nose be your guide when choosing household or other goods that might be capable of adding to your personal pollution level: avoid anything that has more than the slightest plastic smell. And never, never burn plastic products or breathe the fumes from burning plastic.

If you are surrounded by plastic derivatives that fill your air with unavoidable fumes, you may have a serious problem. Some people living in houses or mobile homes with urea-formaldehyde foam insulation have been forced to move or have the insulation removed because they were unable to enjoy a healthy life when they were breathing formaldehyde every day. If you suspect this to be at the root of your problem, you could check your suspicions by going somewhere else for a couple of weeks – ideally somewhere as unpolluted as a stone-built cottage in rural Wales – to see if your condition improves. This isn't a perfect test by any means, but it might give you an insight into your situation.

People living in gas-heated homes, or cooking on gas stoves, have a similar problem. Many allergy sufferers have had all their gas appliances removed and report a considerable improvement in their condition. But this is an expensive choice to make and you will want to be sure that gas is a serious problem for you before you do it. We suggest that you get the gas company to switch your home off for a few weeks in the summer while you rely on electric appliances. If you are sensitive to gas, you should notice a marked change in the way you feel within a few days.

We would advise all those who suffer from persistent fat, or who have any reason to believe their bodies do not cope well with chemicals, to avoid using gas. Bear this in mind when you choose a new home.

Avoiding chemicals can have some potentially annoying consequences. One is the need to adjust to an environment that other creatures can share – a good sign because it is life-supporting.

If flies are not being killed by poisons in the air in your home, then they do tend to buzz around the room! And when you take the flea collar off your pet and throw away the pest spray, you are liable to face flea problems. What should you do?

There is the possibility of changing your own perception a little. We are much less tolerant of other life-forms now we can practise mass-murder by poison. Perhaps the odd insect in the home is not so dreadful?

Other ways of dealing with pests are available, even if they are not as thorough as chemicals can be. The vacuum cleaner was responsible for banishing the human flea from our homes; it is still the most potent weapon. Used frequently, especially where your pet sleeps, it will keep the level of fleas down. Steam-cleaning is marvellous for carpets and upholstery; it will remove pests without harming you or your pet. But most important if you want to minimize fleas: don't let your pets wander through the whole house and sleep on your bed.

There are three methods of coping with flies (apart from encouraging spiders – the true bio-slut's answer!). First, family fun with fly swats; some people are more efficient with these than others. (Confirmed bio-sluts will let ants tidy the remains away.) Second, hang sticky fly paper from the ceiling – but don't let your hair brush against it. Third, there's the non-chemical electronic insect repeller used in food shops.

Doing It Yourself around the home can also create real difficulties for the PFR sufferer. There's no point working to detoxify your system and rebuild your liver if you are being exposed to doses of chemicals that could undo all your re-constructive work in a couple of days. And the sort of chemicals we use as handypersons are very often potent liver poisons.

As with household products, the best guide to the potential danger of any substance you are using is your nose. Solvents often have a strong smell. While they will not all be equally dangerous to you, you may not know which ones to avoid until damage has occurred. It's far wiser to recognize that all of them will put a load on your detoxifying systems, and avoid them whenever you can.

This will mean that you will have to stop doing certain household jobs unless you can take the work outdoors and stay upwind of any fumes. Glueing, varnishing, wood preserving, painting (except with water-based paints), paint-stripping and cleaning brushes can be extremely hazardous in confined spaces.

Often, your body will help you to identify those chemicals which are most likely to damage you. Sensitive people tend to become highly aware of the nastiness of solvents. What you must not do is put up with them, reassuring yourself that you won't be painting this door or glueing that piece of furniture for long. The damage occurs more quickly than you realize. In molecular terms it may not need much to trigger your liver into its dumping routine.

So when you want to do these jobs, choose technology that does not involve solvents whenever you can. Remove paint with sandpaper rather than paint-stripper and use screws instead of glue. And if one of your rooms gets contaminated, stay out of it until it's thoroughly aired and smells safe.

Your body may tell you in other ways that something you have encountered is bad for you. A sudden desire for sweet or fat food, or hunger beyond your normal appetite for no obvious reason, are good clues. If you experience this, try to identify the stimulus and avoid it. (Dieters who are always hungry will not get these messages. Another example of how harmful working against your body can be.)

Finally, we cannot leave the subject of the air you breathe in your home without tackling the problem of cigarette smoke. If you are a smoker, you can probably predict some of what we have to say about it, but the reasons may be new to you.

Giving up smoking is an essential part of the PFR Escape Plan. You may be surprised at this, because you will know that people tend to put on weight when they give up smoking. But the Plan is no ordinary way of losing unwanted fat and its principles, although entirely logical, are at variance with many of our usual assumptions.

There are many problems with cigarettes, some of which we describe later in this book. At this point, the important fact is that nicotine is a potent liver poison. In some ways, its effect on the liver is similar to that of DDT – nicotine can actually be used as an insecticide.

There is no way round it; you need to give up. Give up completely. You probably wish you could, just like that, and that there were no unpleasant consequences.

We know the consequences. We are both ex-smokers. We know what it's like to go through withdrawal – and we know that it's not the same for everybody. Perhaps for you it's particularly difficult. Or maybe you haven't been sufficiently convinced of the need to go through with it before.

So how do you give up? There are books which will help with this, and fact packs from Action on Smoking and Health and the Health Education Council. There may be an anti-smoking clinic in your area. Acupuncture helps some people.

First, acknowledge that nicotine is a tranquillizer, and that's why you use it. The strategy we describe in the next chapter will help to reduce your stress level and reduce your desire for nicotine.

Choose a time to give up cigarettes when you do not expect to be under pressure. Set yourself a date and tell yourself, your friends, workmates and family that you will not smoke another cigarette after the date you've chosen. And they are not to do anything that might shake your resolve. Maybe some will join you – it's easier to give up in company with others.

Perhaps you ought to get angry about being a drug addict – angry with yourself, and angry with those commercial and political interests that want to keep you hooked. Accept that you are likely to feel anxious, miserable, unwell. Withdrawal from addictive tranquillizers is almost always unpleasant. But you can do it if you really want.

Avoiding Chemicals at Work
Some cameos illustrate common problems.

Jane was a laboratory technician. She gave up her job after she realized that her blackouts, nausea and depression were associated with exposure to the fume-laden air of her work environment.

Anna works in a modern, air-conditioned office. Everything seems very clean and efficient – but Anna has noticed that she always seems to feel unwell, with headaches and stuffiness, when she's in the office. Most of her colleagues have similar experiences, though the severity of the problem varies.

Judith is a highly trained nurse. She used to work in the operating theatre, handing the instruments to the surgeons, sometimes finishing stitching after surgery. But frequent headaches, nausea and dizziness forced her to return to the wards.

These women are typical of thousands who work in places where the air is contaminated with chemicals which overload their detoxifying systems. Some of the most modern office buildings are known to make so many of their employees ill that a 'sick-building syndrome' has been identified. It is caused by the recirculation of polluted air within these buildings.

When office workers could open windows and get plenty of fresh air to breathe, the main problem was keeping warm enough. Today buildings are heated to midsummer temperatures all the year round, but so that the costs are not prohibitive, opportunities for exchanging air with the chilly outdoors are severely restricted. Under these circumstances, fumes can accumulate in the recycled air.

Sources of fumes in the modern office may not be obvious, but to the sensitive person they can pose a real threat. Old-fashioned photocopiers, carbonless copying paper, solvents used to clean equipment such as typewriters or the disk drives of computers – all these produce fumes. Add optional extras such as nail varnish remover, 'air freshener' and hairspray, and you can end up with a formidable chemical problem.

Places like laboratories and hospitals are very hazardous for anyone whose detoxifying capacity is limited. Solvents used for preserving and staining, antiseptic chemicals and anaesthetics all put a load on the liver. Indeed, some anaesthetists and surgical nurses have developed serious liver disease from frequent exposure to small quantities of these gases.

If you are exposed to chemicals at work, you will be faced with a very difficult decision. Perhaps you love nursing, or you find your job in a chemically polluted air-conditioned office very stimulating or lucrative. You need to decide how seriously the chemical pollution of your workplace threatens you – and how important it is to you to lose that persistent fat. It may be very difficult to do while you keep that job.

It is often possible to reach a compromise. Like Judith, you may be able to move away from the worst problems while staying in the same line of work. Or you may be able to move into an office with a window that you can open. Possibly you will be able to insist on improvements in your workplace which reduce the chemical load – more efficient ventilation is the obvious step.

Some trades unions are very concerned about chemical hazards in the workplace and will represent your case, and those of others like you, to the management. It could well be worthwhile talking about it.

All of this may seem to present an impossibly large task. Do not be put off. Remember that what you are searching for are the particular things that are adversely affecting you. Because there are so many possibilities and such variation between people, it is impossible for us to say 'avoid this, or that, and you will be fine'. We just can't tell what is causing your problem, so we have to give very broad guidance.

Take a patient, long-term view. Listen to your body and your instincts; as you lower your general loading of pollution, you will become more sensitive to particular things. Clearing away some of the load will cause the culprits to emerge. When this happens, follow your hunches – have confidence in yourself.

Of course, it would be wonderful if the world were a clean and natural place, fit for humans to live in without these problems. Changes are happening, but they take time. You can help –

indeed, you already are. By eating good pure food and cleaning up your personal world, you are helping to make it better for all of us. Keep up the good work – you have nothing to lose but that unwanted fat!

CHAPTER 12

Mobilize Your Metabolism

Warning: You should not attempt to follow the later recommendations in this chapter until you have established the eating pattern described in chapter 10 (Schedule 1) and significantly reduced your environmental toxin loading as described in the last chapter. To do so could make your PFR problem worse.

Remember this is an integrated plan; all parts of it are important and must be carried out in the correct sequence. Check the week-by-week action plan (chapter 13) if you are in any doubt.

Mobilizing your metabolism has three phases, each with a different emphasis, but each one part of a complementary sequence. The objectives of these phases can be summarized as recovery, running in and revving up.

The first objective is fairly straightforward, but for many people its requirements can be all too elusive. It involves the equivalent of convalescence: eating well and getting adequate rest so that the natural recuperative powers of the body can operate.

The second requires the addition of a pattern of foundation activity. This will prepare you for the final part of the Plan.

The final objective is to encourage your body to build on its foundation of recovery and basic activity. This involves eating and activity patterns that will increase your liver capacity. With this enhanced capacity you will go on to mobilize your persistent fat in a safe and natural way. The establishment of this lifestyle is the final stage in getting rid of persistent fat – and keeping it off!

First Phase

The first phase of the Plan starts with good rest. Rest is essential for recovery and regeneration. When you are asleep, your body switches off its activity functions and concentrates instead on repairing daytime wear and tear, rebuilding long-term damage and restructuring to meet future needs.

What you must do is ensure that you are getting enough rest. It is essential that you get a good night's sleep every night. If anything is preventing you achieving this, you must regard it as a major problem and solve it.

If it is a matter of bad habits, you can easily change them. Too much coffee in the evening, or being overstimulated before going to bed, are common problems. Change your routine, begin winding down earlier. Close down the stimulation or demands which are making you restless. Relaxing music, a book at bedtime, sex, a hot bath, a short stroll – make sure you get whatever will help get you into a state where you can sleep deep and well.

If your problem is made worse by light, noise or other people, take action. Turn it off, shut it out, or make them go away. Invest in comfortable ear plugs, heavy, lined curtains or sound-proofing. The improvement, both in your environment and in you, could be tremendous.

It may be that the way your life is structured means that such simple changes are not enough. If your routine is geared to servicing the needs of others: up to get husband or children off in the morning, the housework or job-filled day, and care, comfort and companionship in the evenings, you have got to change it. The answer is to be selfish.

Look carefully at where your time and effort is going. Is it really essential that you do so much for others? Women can easily slip into habits of living their lives for and through others. Part of your escape from PFR is to get in control of your body; to do this you must establish some control over your life. Change the terms of your relationships with those around you; tell them why you are doing it, and enlist their help. Your objective is to get time on your side so that you can rest and recuperate. It is crucial that you reduce any factors that may be putting you under stress. This is because our whole reaction to stress is the very opposite of what we are trying to achieve with adequate rest and recuperation. Chronic stress goes so far the other way that it actually induces serious illness such as heart disease and ulcers. So it is important to resolve any problems which are generating stress in your life, particularly if you know that they cause a state of chronic stress.

The general key to stress management is to reduce causes and build up your ability to cope. The later parts of the Plan will do this as an added bonus, but for now you may have to pause and concentrate on reduction. There are many books which can help; our own *The Long-Life Heart: How to Avoid Heart Disease and Live a Longer Life* will help you both assess and manage stress factors. You may need to consult your doctor (do not take drugs, either for stress or to help with sleep) or perhaps to look for specialist counselling.

It may be that some of your wind-down time could be spent removing stress. Many people find that specialized relaxation techniques like meditation or yoga are very helpful. If these appeal to you, now is the time to follow up your interest. It is usually best to get proper instruction; find a teacher or join a class and get expert training in the method you choose.

You can start to prime your system once you have established a routine that copes with stress and ensures you are getting enough sleep – and that means as much as you need, ignore other peoples' standards! Wake up feeling rested and have a nap in the day if you feel like it. This will aid recuperation and get you ready to mobilize that fat.

Your liver needs as much oxygen as it can get for detoxification and regeneration. You may think that because breathing is automatic, you will get as much as you need without making any special effort. This is often not so, but if you decide on yoga or meditation, controlled breathing which adds to your oxygen intake could be a valuable part of your routine.

This is another reason why we stressed giving up smoking in the previous chapter. Not only is it very direct personal pollution, but it reduces your oxygen-carrying capacity. When you smoke, you inhale the nicotine that keeps you hooked, and also carbon monoxide. This combines with the pigment in the red corpuscles of your blood, the haemoglobin, to form carboxyhaemoglobin, which is resistant to breakdown. By doing this, the carbon monoxide prevents the haemoglobin doing what it should – carrying oxygen from your lungs. Cigarette smokers can reduce their oxygen-carrying capacity by up to 20 per cent in this way.

Even if you are not a smoker, years of tension, bad posture or a sedentary lifestyle cause many people to adopt breathing patterns that do not get as much oxygen as they need into their system. If you ever feel breathless or have panic attacks, this could be the cause. Back to yoga for breathing exercises.

Everyone should follow a simple breathing routine, at least three times a day, to help oxygenate the body. Below is a routine that can be followed anywhere. Once a day before you start a breathing session, check your posture. This is important simply to get your rib cage into the right shape, to take restrictive pressure off your lungs and to let the whole breathing system work properly.

Stand as tall as you can, with your back against a wall or other flat surface. Try to get your heels, calves and buttocks against the wall. Then as you breathe in, push your shoulders back and stretch your head up as tall as you can. Breathe in and out three times very slowly and deeply, pushing your shoulders back and head up each time. You may feel a little faint, or your heart may knock. Don't worry, it's just the unaccustomed oxygen and the pressure you have taken off.

Try to keep that shoulders-back, head-up posture. Think how good it is for your heart. The breathing routine can be done sitting, preferably on a firm chair, or on the floor. With your back in the new posture, think carefully about what you are doing, and breathe in very slowly, as slowly as you can. As your lungs fill and your ribs rise, think about what is happening inside, relate the feeling to the reality. When your lungs are full, try to squeeze in a little more, push your belly out to lower your diaphragm. When you are full up, hold it as long as you can; then reverse the process, diaphragm then ribs, and empty your lungs. Hold the empty position as long as you can, then repeat. Do it at least ten times – more if you want a meditative high that is entirely natural!

At first it may be difficult to time your effort through a whole breathing cycle. Practice will get it right. And it will be quite hard work, but you will feel the supercharging effects fairly quickly. Do it any time you want to calm down or prime yourself to accomplish a difficult task.

First Phase objectives
Establish a routine that gives you plenty of sleep, ensures you can rest when necessary, and that you are not living under continual stress.

Then build in your regular breathing routine every day.

You can link the parts together to suit yourself so that they complement each other. A positive pattern will start to emerge.

Second Phase
While maintaining your established rest and breathing routines, the time has now come to build some activity into your life. Keep your diet pattern on that given in Schedule 1 (chapter 10) and if you want to eat more as your activity level increases, go with it. Trust your body, eat when you are hungry. You need plenty of good food, both for continuing recuperation, and for the activity you are going to be doing.

This activity is a foundation. It is a basic minimum intended to get your systems turning over – something like running a car in before you start to use it. Take your time through this stage –

keep those rest and breathing patterns going.

Do not worry if you are not very physical at the present. Most people who have had PFR for years will be out of condition and probably only just managing with the daily routine. Start from where you are; you will rapidly improve as all the parts of the Plan begin to affect your condition for the better. If you really need absolute beginners' help read Appendix 4; the basic movement is basic enough to get anyone started.

While we are discussing getting started, let's deal with common blocks: thoughts like 'I can't do that sort of thing', 'I will feel silly' and so on. Forget it, everyone is capable of moving and becoming slim and fit. For some it will be a longer journey than for others. Even if you have never thought it possible, one step at a time will get you there. Just make up your mind to take the first step. Remember the end of the journey is a permanently thinner you.

Enjoy yourself! When you start being active on the Plan, whatever you do, make it fun. If you are miserable, you are fighting your body again. At times it will be hard, but it should still be enjoyable – we will suggest ways which will help.

And get the right clothes. If you are a beginner, do not try to manage without the right clothes. Basics which everyone should have are: a pair of good trainers with solid but padded soles, the sort used by runners. And suitable clothing; this should be minimal, wear just enough to keep you warm. A cotton track suit with shorts and a running vest is the aim, but initially something light and loose that allows free movement. You may also need a specialized sports bra. Remove other sources of distraction. Take off jewellery and do not worry about hair or make-up. Time for all that later; when you are being active, be single-minded and be yourself.

Good, comfortable and well-fitting footwear is essential, particularly if your feet are carrying a heavy load or have been distorted by too many years in high heels. Go to a specialist sports shop. No matter how 'un-sporty' you are now, you are moving in that direction, so start off as you mean to go on. Do not make the mistake of sliding into the fashion shop out of embarrassment or for the pretty colours. That is fashion sports wear. It is for posers who are not serious. Do not be shy – sports shops are usually staffed by enthusiasts who will want to help and encourage you. And if you have never had a pair of good trainers before, you will have a pleasant surprise. We know a seventy-year-old couple (now doing ten-mile sponsored walks) who said it was like having new feet!

A word of caution: if at any time after an activity session you experience feelings of hangover or nausea, it means you have done too much. Wait two or three days, then try again. This time do about half as much as before. If this goes well, build up gradually; even if you feel physically capable of more, your metabolism may not be up to it yet. Patience!

In this second phase, activity is essential to bring your systems up to par. In a real sense it is the continuation of the rest and recuperation regime described above. It is not for removing fat, although that may happen incidentally. The aim is not strenuous activity, strain, stiffness or sweat, just a gentle build up to our basic objective. Once achieved, you will be in a position to start on the last lap – shedding that toxic adipose tissue permanently.

What you should aim to achieve is this: a period of brisk walking for about half an hour, covering a minimum of two miles, each day. This means continuous walking, not stopping. You should be doing it every day for at least two weeks with no problems before you consider moving on to the next phase.

Now, for some people that will be easy; others will find it a long way off. Whatever your ability, the old familiar question of having the time is the most likely first barrier. Take it, or make it! You are approaching the point where you can say goodbye to that weight, don't sink back now.

If you are so overweight or out of condition that this is not possible, do not despair. The activities in Appendix 4 will start you off; when you combine this with other parts of the Plan and increased energy output in your daily routine, you will soon be there. Take your time and keep the rest of the Plan going.

For everyone else, time to get your trainers on. Add some suitable and comfortable clothes and set off. Do not worry if you cannot walk far at first; do what you comfortably can. Remember brisk minutes are better than sloppy hours, so sing a bouncy tune in your head and stride off to it. Breathe deep as you go, shoulders back, loose but purposeful. Aim for steady co-ordinated rhythm, swing your arms, and keep the momentum up so that it carries you along.

Measure your time at first. Once you can walk continuously for thirty minutes, measure the distance you can cover, either with a map or with a car speedometer. Check out some other routes while you are about it so you can vary your scenery.

When you come back, even if you are only out for minutes, give yourself a reward. Athletes and sportspersons have a whole wind-down routine, with a shower or bath and relaxation period. Why not you? It does not have to be anything in particular, just something you like that gives you pleasure – a little self-spoiling will encourage your efforts.

Once you have got your time-slot established and are on the way to achieving two miles in half an hour or less, you might like to vary your activity. How about half an hour on a bike? You go a lot further, but the breathing and the rhythmic movement are what you should aim for. Or go swimming, but watch out for adverse effects from chlorinated water.

Now you can start to be more adventurous: perhaps regular energetic dancing. You are on the way to being slim and healthy, so you might as well start practising the sort of habits that go with a slim and healthy lifestyle! Throughout all your activity listen to your body, keep feeling the air flowing in and out, try to sense in your mind exactly how your muscles are moving – locate their control circuits and play with them. Tense and relax; make your limbs move the way you want them to. Stretch and contract; feel the range you are capable of. And enjoy all the sensations of being in control!

How long do you need to maintain the foundation activity?

What you are actually doing is rebuilding yourself, getting your body, your habits and your attitudes back into order, so as long as you are enjoying it, carry on. If you are getting restless, think about whether you are ready for the next phase. It is important not to start until you are absolutely ready. False starts are very unnerving.

It takes as long as it takes, but some rough guide can be given. The crucial thing is the state of your liver. For those under thirty who were not terribly overweight or inactive, three to six weeks should be reasonable. For those between thirty and fifty in the same condition, say four to eight weeks. Those older or with more ground to make up may take a lot longer. Can you carry out your half an hour of activity every day without any signs of distress?

The best indication that you are ready to move on is a stable feeling of increased general health, increased energy and clear-headedness. Watch out for false positives caused by hormone shifts in the female monthly cycle. By now you will know yourself a lot better than when you started on the Plan, and you are your best guide. If you feel ready, and vibrantly confident, then go!

Third Phase

In this third and final phase we will be using activity to mobilize your remaining persistent fat. At this point we must sound another warning: if you are pregnant or breastfeeding, the final phase is not yet for you. Stay with the second phase but take longer walks as you get fitter. Start on the final phase when your baby's weaned.

As you move into phase three, you should start changing your eating pattern to Schedule 2 (chapter 10). Change your eating routine gradually as you start activities that will mobilize your rebuilt liver and finally rid your body of the toxins which are locking that fat in place.

A changed pattern of physical activity is essential because it is the only way to persuade the liver to mobilize those fat stores.

What you have to do is this: three hours after the last meal of the day, undertake enough activity to run down the liver's glycogen stores; then go to bed. While you sleep your liver will recharge – not from food – but from your fat. It is as simple as that.

It is important to realize that as you persuade your system to lose its final deposits of toxic adipose tissue, two things may happen. First, your body may lose other fat in preference to contaminated tissue, and second, it may still try to replace fat. Both are indications that the toxins locked up are presenting problems.

You should be prepared to allow your body to make some more fat. Your system may be using it to dilute the toxins already stored; when they are at an acceptable level, it will metabolize them. So for this first stretch of the last lap, make sure those meals are big enough! Your body is adding another task to its recuperative and activity loading: it now has to act to detoxify itself. Hunger is your body telling you it has a problem dealing with the fat you are trying to mobilize and you should not try to override it. But this doesn't mean you should stuff yourself with food when you know you don't need it.

In addition to the problem of releasing and metabolizing toxins, you will also have to be alert to other transitory problems which may occupy your liver capacity. Minor infections or other illness may cause reduced energy or exhaustion. If this happens, ease off; do not further overload the system. When you have recovered from the infection, press ahead again.

Warning: If the level and pattern of activity you are now embarking on produces any hangover effects, you must reduce your activity level. If they persist, you must go back to the previous phase. You are obviously not ready for the last lap, and if you go on, you risk the possibility of serious damage to your other organs. It will not solve the PFR problem because your metabolism is clearly not yet able to cope.

You have become accustomed to a gentle daily activity routine;

now you need to speed it up. You know where your local sports shop is: get a good track suit. Have whatever colour you like, but get one that is predominantly cotton. In summer you need a fairly light one; in winter a heavy warm one.

This is the pattern of activity you need to follow.

Three times a week, with a gap of at least one day in between – say Monday, Wednesday and Friday – you should spend thirty to forty-five minutes on strenuous activity which will cause your liver to burn up its glycogen stores.

Glycogen is used up under the influence of adrenalin, so the activity needs to be violent enough to get your heart rate up, make you sweat and keep you on the edge of breathlessness. Sounds like fun? During your period of strenuous activity you should not ease off enough to stop sweating, just enough to get your breath back when necessary to allow you to continue.

The body stores energy at many levels. Most of our ordinary activity just uses local energy stored in the muscles. In order to persuade your liver that you are serious, and need it to start discharging its glycogen, you have to use up these local stores. 'Second wind' is the phenomenon of feeling exhausted and then suddenly discovering new energy; the exhaustion is when the local energy is gone, and the renewed energy is when the liver does its stuff.

Once you have completed this activity, wind down, bathe, relax, drink some water or diluted fruit juice, and go straight to bed. On the days you are not doing this, continue your breathing and relaxation. Your metabolism will still be working away for you – if you pushed it hard enough to use up that glycogen.

Don't be alarmed at the violent effects of such physical activity. Many of the things we do for fun produce these effects! Dancing routines, running, brisk hill walking, weight training, hard cycling and rowing, all produce this reaction and are all suitable. So are some traditional activities, like sawing logs, heavy digging, lawn mowing without a motor-mower – a lot of the things we used to do in the days before PFR was a problem for so many people.

You can use aerobic-type exercise, or dance exercise routines, to achieve the same effect. Whatever you do, it must be something you can work at continuously for at least half an hour. Stop-start sports like squash are not suitable; your liver will only turn on through continuous demand – this is why athletes involved in such sports warm up first, to turn their liver glycogen on so that the energy is instantly available.

There is one possible problem you must be aware of: the activity plateau. As you push yourself, your capacity will increase – it will seem easier. It is easy to get into a routine where you do the same amount each time, but as your capacity has increased, this becomes a smaller percentage of what you are capable of, or what you need to do. You will have settled on a stable plateau. One way to avoid this is to vary your activity; go running on Mondays, cycling on Wednesdays, and so on. Don't let yourself settle into a dull routine.

The rate at which you use energy during activity will be rather low at first. It will build up as your liver gets used to the idea and builds more capacity. This is the wonderful thing about physical activity; the more you do, the more you can do. One day you will look at yourself and wonder where that feeble, flabby person has gone. The new you will be a source of wonder, pleasure and pride. When you feel that, you are on the home straight. PFR will be a thing of the past, as will everything that goes with it.

Running is one of the best activities we know for tuning up the liver. But you should not start running before you can walk efficiently! Your phase two foundation should have got you to the point where you are ready; check your performance with this simple test, it will tell you whether you are ready to start running.

Note your starting time; then walk two miles on level ground as briskly as you can. Do not stop. How long did it take you?

If you took more than thirty minutes, you need to do more fast walking. Similarly, if you had to stop because of leg pain, you need more practice. You are not ready for phase three yet!

Carry on walking every day, increase the speed you go and the distance you cover. If you took between twenty-five and thirty minutes, start doing some yards of trotting every few minutes during your walk. Gradually build up the speed and distance you are trotting. If you took less than twenty-five minutes, you are ready to start running. Warm up with an exercise routine such as the Canadian Air Force system described in *Physical Fitness* (Recommended Reading, p. 184). Then go out and run! Non-runners should start reading about technique, or ask a runner friend for help; many people, especially women, simply don't know how to run, and until they learn the right type of movement they're not likely to enjoy it. And as you are well on the way to being a physically competent, athletic person, take some time off and watch the pros on television; see how they move. Look particularly at people whose skeletal build is like yours. If you would prefer, watch dancers or other performers. You can learn a lot by observing the way they move.

Do choose your running route with an eye to the pollution levels you'll encounter! Avoid all busy roads, keep to paths and parks as much as you can. When you're breathing in all the air you need to keep on running, you don't want to be taking in great quantities of exhaust fumes. The same goes for cycling routes.

Throughout your activity, control your breathing; this is particularly important when running. Breathe as slowly as you can, use the control you have learned earlier. Fast panting won't deliver as much oxygen as long, slow breaths. Try counting as you stride – in, two, three, out, two, three. It should come together as an integrated whole, your breathing, striding and heart rate. This stable expression of energy over a period of time is stamina.

Push off from your toes, reach forward with your leg, and land on your heel. The foot rolls with each step. Aim for an easy, economical movement; stretch your legs and vary your length of stride as you go.

Never push yourself too hard or too long. If you feel any pain anywhere (apart from the nag of tired muscles), then rest. Don't struggle through any pain barriers. In that way people injure themselves and put themselves off running – it's totally counter-productive and very foolish. You must not be a martyr to your exercise routine.

And do not neglect to reward yourself when you get back. A hot bath or shower will be essential now. How about a luxurious massage afterwards – your partner should oblige as a con-tribution towards your efforts. Keep thinking of special treats. There will come a time when what you are actually doing is its own reward. If this happens, you are hooked. You are now a confirmed physical animal, and will just enjoy being physical!

For those who do not want to run, there are alternatives. Hard cycling can have excellent effects; also dancing (leaping and throwing yourself about energetically – remember Mick Jagger? None of that foot shuffling that could exhaust nobody!) You can do it at home to your favourite records. Aerobics and dancing can be good, and games like tennis and football are fine, but only if you're an energetic player, playing hard, fast and continuously.

When you are doing any form of strenuous activity, you will notice the signs of increased liver activity. After a few minutes of muscular work, you start to feel warm, you'll peel off a couple of layers of clothing. That's the first sign – the liver controls your body temperature, and it's adjusting to changing con-ditions. If you carry on, you'll start feeling tired; but when you experience your second wind, you'll find you can go on much further than you thought initially. That's the sign of the next increment in liver activity, injecting sugar into your blood-stream from its glycogen stores.

Sometimes, you'll experience a less pleasant sign: pain, rather like stitch, on the right hand side of your body. Unlike classic stitch, this occurs when you haven't had a meal for three hours or more before your activity began. If you slow down, rest a bit and then continue, the pain disappears, and you find you have more energy. That may be the liver injecting nutrients into your bloodstream.

Make sure you get enough rest and recuperate sufficiently after each session of demanding activity. It is essential that you maintain yourself in excellent health so that your detoxifying capacity continues to grow.

Keep up this routine and your fat will gradually disappear. Remember to avoid the hangover zone of over-activity, but every once in a while do a little more than usual, see if you still have toxins in your system.

You may want to do less strenuous activities on alternate days. Be guided by the signals from your body; if you are sure you can cope with walking, cycling or other activities on the days between your strenuous work-outs, then go ahead. It will help keep your systems loose and speed up the loss of fat.

What about your weight? Throughout the Plan you have been replacing unhealthy tissue with uncontaminated fat and healthy muscle, and on the last lap you have been reducing the fat content. Your body should now have a minimal amount of fat, and a lot of healthy tissue. You may actually be heavier, but – back to your mirror – isn't your shape much better?

You are also in control of your body; you have learned a new way of eating as much healthy food as you need, and how to protect yourself against potential hazards in your environment. You are now in a position to decide what sort of body shape you would like for the rest of your life. Chapter 14 tells you how to get and keep it.

To start on the Plan you will find all the recommendations brought together in week-by-week action summaries in the following chapter. Now that you have digested the information you will be able to use these charts as a practical action guide.

CHAPTER 13

Week-by-Week Action Plan

This chapter is for guidance. You must adapt the time-scale to suit your personal needs. Don't stick rigidly to our suggestions – because they were designed for the hypothetical 'average reader' and you won't be that person – she doesn't actually exist. Base your personal Plan on our time-scale, taking particular note of the sequence of actions, and missing no steps on the way, but monitor your own progress and give yourself more time if you need it.

Throughout the early weeks it is important that you keep looking at yourself, and that you keep your self-esteem up. Remember what you are working towards; start thinking and behaving like the sort of person you are going to be.

Your escape from PFR should be seen as an exploratory and joyful journey into a new way of life. There will be adventures and difficulties but it should be seen from the outset as the most rewarding period of your life. Enjoy the experience and have fun along the way!

Week 1

Theme: discovery and analysis
Major tasks: identify pollutants
                record established lifestyle

In the first week you should start keeping a detailed diary. This will follow on from the notes you have been making of things particularly relevant to you from the last three chapters. Record the forces that are acting on you now and which may be responsible for maintaining your PFR problem. Look at all the aspects of your life that we highlighted in chapters 10 to 12.

DIET

Record the food you eat each day, including any snacks. Record the quantities you have and note how many of your food sources could cause pollution problems. Note which foods and drinks you think you could not give up easily – you could be addicted to these. How often do you normally consume them? Are you 'topping up' at regular intervals?

REST

Note how much total rest you get. How much of your relaxation time is spent alone? Are you able to relax deeply when you've stopped working? How many hours are you sleeping? Can you identify anything that interferes with your sleep?

Note when you feel tired or sleepy. When does this happen? Is it associated with eating meals or particular foods or with long gaps between meals? Are you able to rest when you feel tired?

ACTIVITY

How far do you walk (or cycle) each day? How often do you use the car? Do you drive when there's no real need?

ENVIRONMENTAL POLLUTION

Go through the questionnaire (p. 115) to determine the pollution level in your home. What are the major sources? Start discarding air pollutants such as insecticides, 'air fresheners' and sprays.

Smokers: record the number of cigarettes you smoke, and

when you smoke them. What are the circumstances that induce smoking?

Those who work away from home: check potential sources of pollution in your work environment. Record all you find in a week.

APPRAISAL

At the end of the week, look at the information you've gathered about yourself. You're already gaining insight into the nature of your personal problem – and that's a big step towards solving it.

Week 2

Theme: preparation
Major tasks: removing pollutants

In the second week, you will use the knowledge gained in Week 1 to begin reducing some of the worst hazards in your environment. At the same time, you should focus on the sources of personal stress in your life that could be undermining your coping systems.

DIET

Find suppliers of organic wholefoods, buy basic supplies of YES foods. Phase out high-additive foods. Start sprouting mung beans and grains such as wheat. Invest in new cookbooks if necessary; experiment with ways of preparing food that will fit in with the PFR diet.

REST

If you have been having problems getting as much rest or sleep as you want, start looking at them. Try building naps into your day – perhaps in the afternoon or mid-evening. Give up drinking coffee after 5pm.

If your relaxation problems are associated with stress, plan how to deal with the major causes. Find help (counsellors, yoga teachers, support groups) if appropriate. Give yourself plenty of time to solve these problems – but start working on them for positive change.

MEDICATION

Medication users should find out about alternative methods of dealing with their problems. Discuss phasing out your drugs with your doctor. The comments on stress, above, may be relevant. Your lifestyle changes in future weeks will help.

Pill-users should explore barrier methods of contraception (diaphragm, sheath) or the possibility of sterilization.

ACTIVITY

Start your deep breathing routine. Buy some good trainers and start wearing them in.

ENVIRONMENTAL POLLUTION

List the hazards you're going to eliminate first. Work out how to manage without them; acquire substitutes if necessary. Work through your list, crossing them off one by one.

Smokers start planning when you'll give up. Investigate stress-reduction methods if you think you'll need them.

Identify hazards at work, seek ways to reduce them.

Week 3

Theme: detoxification
Major task: removing pollutants

DIET

Get established on the PFR diet (Schedule 1). Continue sprouting beans, seeds, etc. What else can you grow yourself? Check out seed displays in garden shops for inspiration if you haven't grown your own before; invest in a book on organic gardening. If you believe you're allergic to some of the YES foods, start the diet without them, but always ensure you're eating comparable foods in equivalent quantities. For example, you may want to substitute rice and millet for wheat, or nuts and seeds for eggs.

Note any withdrawal symptoms you experience with your changed diet. You could be allergic to the foods or drinks you most crave. Don't give in – give it time. You will feel much better after a week.

REST

Continue to ensure that you get plenty of sleep.

ACTIVITY

Continue your deep breathing routine. Take a daily walk, two miles at a steady, brisk pace. If this is too much for you, start building up your stamina with frequent shorter walks. Try the 'Dance' advice in appendix 4.

ENVIRONMENTAL POLLUTION

Initiate action to reduce pollution in your workplace if necessary. Finish removing hazards from your home.

Week 4

Theme: detoxification
Major task: liver regeneration

DIET

You should be eating five small meals a day, drawn from the

YES group of foods.

Give up tea, coffee and alcohol completely; substitute spring water, diluted fruit juices, vegetable juices, herb teas and/or dandelion coffee.

Make sure you have sufficient sprouts for each day – vary the seeds, beans, etc. Try different types such as alfalfa, wheat, sunflower. Eat some raw cashew nuts, brazil nuts and/or sunflower seeds daily.

Some women may wish to add evening primrose oil as a dietary supplement – especially during the second half of the monthly cycle. Vitamin B6 may also be helpful for those who have pre-menstrual problems which might cause yearnings for chocolate, etc.

REST

Remember you're still treating yourself as a convalescent. Get as much rest as you need to maximize healing.

Do breathing exercises three times daily.

ACTIVITY

Walk or cycle briskly for half an hour each day.

Weeks 5 to 7

Theme: Health enhancement
Major task: Liver regeneration

DIET

Schedule 1: if you left particular foods out of your diet because of suspected allergy, now is the time to try them out. Introduce them one at a time, no more than one per day. If you react badly to one or more of these foods, don't try it again for two months. Never eat any food to which you have shown signs of allergy more often than twice a week, and then only in small amounts. However, you may find that you are not allergic to the organically produced form of the food you thought you couldn't take. You might have been reacting to the residues in it, and have no problems with uncontaminated forms.

REST

You should have established a regime that ensures that you do not feel tired when you wake in the morning, and that you can nap in the day if need be. If this is proving difficult, find a yoga, autogenics or meditation teacher and learn a technique for deep relaxation.

Continue breathing exercises regularly.

ACTIVITY

Gradually increase the length of your daily walks. Make sure you are walking briskly, with a good upright posture that allows slow, deep breathing. Focus on your muscles as you move. Find new paths in your neighbourhood, explore local parks and woods. Take a longer walk once or twice a week, go swimming or dancing to vary your activity routine.

ENVIRONMENTAL POLLUTION

Have you successfully given up smoking yet? If not, do it now. Help your partner to give up if he/she is polluting the air you breathe.

Weeks 8 to 12

Theme: metabolic enhancement
Major task: liver stimulation

DIET

Schedule 1: you may want to increase your carbohydrate intake (roots and grains) as your activity level rises.

REST

Don't neglect it!

ACTIVITY

Daily rhythmic activity, sufficient to make you feel very warm and increase your heart rate. Add varied activities. Test your walking speed. Are you ready to start gentle running? Push yourself harder – but beware exercise hangovers, infections – don't take it too fast.

Warning: Pregnant or lactating women, elderly people and those with any health problems should not progress past this stage. Stay at this level and burn your excess fat off gradually.

Weeks 13 to 18

Theme: fat mobilization
Major task: increasing your body's oxygen use

DIET

Intermediate between Schedules 1 and 2. Boost carbohydrate intake and eat three meals per day of YES foods, plus snacks as required. Drink plenty of pure water, especially after activity.

REST

This must balance your activity. Make sure you relax after every session. Sleep remains important.

ACTIVITY

Alternate days, thirty to forty-five minutes strenuous activity.

Running is strongly recommended. Make sure you do enough to finish your session thoroughly tired and bathed in sweat. Watch out for exercise 'hangovers' – don't do too much, drop back if you find you have. The warning signs are headaches on waking the morning after strenuous exercise, nausea and general malaise.

Never continue working a sore knee, ankle or joint – there's no need to risk injuring yourself! By now you should be reading health and sports magazines that will give you other ideas and guidance on activity details.

Just do enough gentle activity on 'off' days to keep loose and mobile.

If you feel tired or ill, cut back activity to previous level, but don't stop being physically active – this is what will rev up your metabolism and get that toxic adipose tissue mobilized.

Weeks 19 to 25

Theme: fat mobilization
Major task: enhance liver capacity

DIET

Schedule 2: eat one major meal each day, others much smaller. From three hours before your evening activity session (alternate days) until mid-morning the next day, eat nothing; drink only water, diluted fruit juices or herb tea.

On non-activity days, you can eat in the evening if you feel hungry.

Adjust food intake to match increasing energy use.

REST

Always allow complete recuperation after activity sessions. We are building up now!

ACTIVITY

Alternate days: warm up with stretching, body-bending (Canadian Air Force exercises if you like). Follow warm-up with thirty to forty minutes running or similar strenuous activity. Wind down afterwards with a warm bath or shower and go to bed to relax completely.

Other days: gentle activities only, whatever feels right to you. Some cycling, walking if desired.

Weeks 26 to 40

Theme: refinement

DIET

Schedule 2: you should be able to cope with some formerly forbidden substances such as coffee and your favourite cheeses now, but watch your intake. The YES foods should still form your staple diet.

ACTIVITY

Build in specific activities for problem muscle groups. Twice-weekly sessions of weight-training will build a more desirable body shape. Try to be habitually active – consider a new sport or active hobby or get an allotment that needs digging. Take a long walk or cycle ride (two hours or more) once a week.

Weeks 41 on

DIET

Eat as desired but make sure you keep pollution levels low. Women should have frequent small meals; men should eat less often, but greater quantities. Don't let yourself slip into dangerous dietary habits.

ACTIVITY

To maintain a good body shape, you have to stay very active. Choose the types of activities you prefer, and those that produce the sort of body you think you could achieve. The leanest women are long-distance runners and body-builders – but they train for many hours each week to achieve their shape! In general, the more physically active you are, the slimmer you can expect to be.

ENVIRONMENTAL POLLUTION

Campaign for a less polluted world! Join Friends of the Earth, Greenpeace, other concerned bodies – add your voice to the growing chorus of protest.

Go on to the next chapter, you should be ready for it now!

CHAPTER 14

Permanent Good Shape

When you've got yourself into good shape, you will want to keep it for the rest of your life.

By now, having worked through the Plan, you will know yourself very well. You will have a realistic image of yourself, no need for scales or calorie counters, and diets will be of no interest to you. You will understand how your body is working, what makes it want to put on fat and how you can control it. You should also be a more physically competent and healthier person. We hope that in addition to learning how much activity you need to keep your metabolism at its best, you will also enjoy being active.

You should also be a happier person. In coming to terms with PFR you will have been forced to throw out a lot of those values and beliefs which tend to work for the benefit of others, but against your self-interest. You will have restructured crucial areas of your life to suit your individual needs. Growing awareness of these needs should have convinced you of your value as an individual; the control you now have over your body and your life is a very positive thing. From here you can go on to further fulfilment and achievement as you wish. You have, after all, solved the problems which are major preoccupations and stumbling blocks for most people.

Not only are you well on the way to being an expert in that most important subject, yourself, but you will also be wiser about the ways of the world. You should be looking with new eyes at innovations in food and chemical products. Your suspicion of their potential effects will be based on your personal experience.

The general state of the environment will also be in your mind. You may now see that, just as we cannot pollute the food we eat without harming ourselves, so we cannot pollute the world in general without causing harm.

So avoiding PFR and staying slim involves maintaining a positive life dynamic on many levels. You will have to eat wholesome food for the rest of your life – nothing wrong with that. You will have to keep your personal loading of potential toxins as low as possible. Providing you avoid the substances which prompt your system to create fat, how much weight you carry will be up to you.

The key to success is simple. If you want to be slim, beautiful and energetic, you have to live the life of a slim, beautiful and energetic person. If you live in any other way, you will become a reflection of that lifestyle. Before your understanding of the PFR Syndrome, this would have been a meaningless statement and an unattainable ideal. Now you know what has been happening to you, it is quite realistic.

Having mastered PFR, some of the old rules start to make a little sense again. Providing you eat innocent food, excess calories will tend to be stored in fat for energy. Activity will tend to mobilize any excess fat. But you will always be at risk of PFR and you cannot simply drop back into your old ways – that was where the problem was in the first place.

Your understanding of the functions of fat on your body will allow you to see why you are carrying what you are. You can adjust your lifestyle, its pace and tempo, to choose your place on the fat scale we used in chapter 3.

In the long term, women should adjust their eating pattern to a more essentially female one. They should be mainly vegetarian nibblers, eating from hour to hour whatever they need for their immediate needs. In this way that minimal subcutaneous layer should not be activated too often, either to store energy or discharge it. Because of the smaller female liver, women's energy needs are best met on a current account basis; unlike men, they are not designed to eat widely spaced, large meals. Men and women are different in many ways other than purely sexually; understanding this and eating accordingly will help you avoid some weight pitfalls.

There will be a delicate, and individual, balance between the amount you can eat and the size of your fat reserves. As an ex-PFR sufferer, you must ensure at all times that you eat enough food. Adjust to any surplus by increasing your daily activity levels. This is the only method which will work for you, and for anyone else for that matter; if you attempt passive weight loss, you are heading for trouble. Your body will start losing lean tissue again, with the possibility of tipping you back into PFR. Where that point is is entirely unpredictable. It depends on too many variables. So play safe, eat enough good organic food, don't go hungry and adjust your weight by changing your activity levels.

This applies to all ages. As we grow older, our metabolism tends to slow down, and this means that we can manage with less food. But eating less means you must be extra vigilant about the quality of your food and about environmental pollutants. And, perversely, it may also mean that you have to be more active to keep in shape. Ballerinas, who have to keep super-fit and shapely, find that as they pass their twenties, they have to put more and more work into keeping 100 per cent in shape for their career. Realistically, we are not aiming for this, but the principle behind it will still operate for a lot of people.

Keeping in shape through an active life has two advantages. First you will be a naturally healthier person; after a little while living like this you will be amazed at how feeble those around you seem. Your liver and detoxification systems will be dealing with all those minor infections that afflict people all the time, without you noticing; you just won't catch all those things that are around. And the likelihood of your suffering major conditions, from heart disease to cancer, will be much reduced.

Second, you can decide on the sort of body shape you want to have. Within the limits of your skeletal structure, and the influence of your hormones – which you in turn influence – you can shape your body to your personal desire. Not only in general terms of slim or more rounded, but also in specifics; more shapely legs, thinner thighs perhaps, or better shoulders. What you want is within your grasp; this is what being in control is all about!

Under that fine layer of healthy fat that gives your body its sexual shaping and smooth surface, your shape is determined by your muscles. Our social values used to lead women to believe that muscles were at best undesirable, and at worst uncouth. Since every movement, from the merest arching of an eyebrow to leaping in the air, depends on our muscles, this view was clearly unrealistic. Fortunately, attitudes are changing, even the most feminine of creatures now understands how important good muscles and good muscle tone are to maintain her desired state.

It will take time and effort. There is no way round this. We evolved to be active creatures and it is only by directing that activity, the detail of the way we move and use our bodies, that we maintain a good shape. This is an essential part of the slim and healthy lifestyle. You are no longer misled by claims for 'food'; if you are tempted by claims for easy ways of keeping in shape, apply the same cynical appraisal you should to all commercial enterprises. Ask who is going to get more shapely: you, or their bank balance?

Similarly, you should read magazine articles which offer the slimming or beauty secrets of the stars with a critical eye. What they don't tell you may be more important than what they do. Raquel Welch put it very honestly and succinctly when asked how she kept her desirable shape – 'I work my butt off.'

Another line which should arouse your suspicion is this: 'the latest scientific research has discovered . . .' Often some minor detail of diet or gadgetry is offered as the universal answer that will allow people to disregard the reality of their nature and emerge unscathed, slim and beautiful, if only they buy the product of this research. We notice, when reviewing this sort of thing, that the people who make the claims never seem to benefit from them in the way that they say you will. They are, if not fat, usually at best running to seed, and hardly athletic. Ignore them, and those stars who may sell them testimonials; if it has only just been discovered, it can hardly have affected their lives in the way they imply.

For muscles, as much as other bodily systems, it is true that, if you don't use them, you will lose them. There are two approaches to keeping in shape, and you will already be aware of the conflict of interests involved. You can live in a way which is basically bad for you, and hope to compensate by adding some sport or exercise on top. Or you can live in a way that is good for you, and top up as required with specific activities or pleasurable pursuits. The Plan you have been following is a bit of a hybrid; it has to work for people with many constraints on their lives.

In the short term it may not matter which approach you follow. However if you opt, or are forced to follow, the former you must understand that your lifestyle will bring diminishing returns. This may be all right for a limited period, while you are young and working for a position, or to achieve specific goals, but you should put a time limit on it. It is easy to drift into trying to live in unsatisfactory ways.

Obviously, if you could structure your life so that all your daily needs for activity were met by the way you lived, this would be ideal. Few of us are in the fortunate position of athletes or other stars. But we can, and should, take every opportunity life offers to change towards it. It is a matter of having the right philosophy and view of your own importance.

Whichever way your life is going, you need to work those muscles. A good regime for basic fitness and figure maintenance can be found in *Physical Fitness*, the system developed for both men and women by the Royal Canadian Air Force. It is a good daily foundation system because it only takes about a quarter of an hour for the routine – half an hour if you have a shower – and because the routines themselves are progressively graduated. This means that you can start at whatever level your weak point puts you at and progressively work up.

There is no reason at all why you should not continue with the activities you started while working through the Plan. You could follow them and take up some sport you may have long fancied. Skiing perhaps? Energetic summer days on the tennis courts? Or both, why not? If you do take up a sport, bear in mind what the Wimbledon stars say; they don't play tennis to keep fit, they have to keep fit to play tennis. If you do follow a particular sport, it will add to your fitness, but not necessarily be doing enough to maintain it.

For specific body shaping the rules are fairly straightforward. If you want thin thighs or a flat stomach, shapely buttocks or a firm bosom, or whatever, you have to find an exercise routine that works the muscle groups in the problem area. Once this routine has reduced the overburden of unwanted bulk, you can then decide whether to add more firm shape with more muscle, or to reduce the muscle bulk, fining down, without replacing it with fat.

To increase bulk, perhaps improve the shaping of your calves or shoulders, you need slow movements with a high resistance and a low number of movement repetitions. Weight training is the best method; make sure you warm up completely first, and combine it with your other activities. Do not try to use weight training as a substitute.

If, on the other hand, you wish to reduce the size of a particular muscle group, you need faster movements, lower resistance and higher numbers of repetitions. There are many specialized sources of advice for this sort of body-building. It should be easy to find activity routines which, combined with your self-expertise, will achieve the desired end.

Before you turn into Superwoman, you should take a look at the context of your life. We have found that many people who embark on a campaign to improve their lives are both surprised at the degree to which they succeed, and unprepared for that success.

The main problem area is with personal relationships. If you are steaming away to become slim and athletic, and your partner stays where he is, it is quite possible that you will grow apart. You are after all becoming a different person. To escape PFR you are changing your lifestyle and life dynamic in many ways, some subtle, some obvious, but all will have an effect. If you are married and have a family, there could be problems if you don't anticipate and plan ahead.

The ideal would be to take your partner and your children with you into a new and better future. This will be possible if you treat PFR, and your determination to stay slim and healthy, as a shared project. They may not be PFR victims – but the Plan is not only specific to that condition, it will improve the health and vitality of anyone. And taking the pollution out of their lives may be a necessary part of doing the same for your own. So if you could all work on it together as a family unit, everyone would benefit.

If you are free and single, there may not be problems of this sort. In fact, for you, escaping the PFR Syndrome and setting your life on a more positive and dynamic course is likely only to be beneficial. Nevertheless, you will be changing over a period of time, and you should be aware of the potential impact on your life.

Women should watch out for men becoming insecure. If you have transformed yourself from an unhappy blob into a lithe and competent person before his eyes, he may not be able to cope with the new you. Of course, at many levels he will be pleased, but at some levels he will be worried; will he be able to maintain the balance of your relationship that he was used to? It is likely that the answer will be no. And probably quite rightly so, because there may have been some degree of complicity with your previous state. But you should be able to build something more positive from your new position; you may have to take a bit more of the initiative and exercise more power within your relationship than you have been accustomed to.

In effect, you will have become a younger, more vibrant person. If you have a stable relationship, it is better if you can make those sorts of journeys together. Don't worry about the children; they will think it great if you are joining in more of their games and sports, instead of being one of those prematurely old young mums, always watching from the sidelines. Life is for living, not watching!

For long-term health it is important that you get yourself into a balanced way of life, a stable routine which suits you. And use your new awareness to spread the idea that health for everyone is a balanced relationship between us and the rest of the biosphere – the health of the person is the health of the planet. Maintaining this balance is the key to permanent good shape, to permanent good health and to a long and enjoyable life.

The Rest of the Iceberg

This book has concentrated on the problem of unwanted fat caused by toxins in our diet and environment. We christened this problem the PFR Syndrome but, as you will have gathered, it is possible that PFR is simply the identifiable part of a range of other interrelated problems. What follows is largely speculative – we have no hard evidence to back up the hypotheses we are putting forward. They are intuitive if you like – but they fit the facts.

That persistent fat which we find so irksome is actually a protective mechanism, shielding our bodies from other possible effects of the substances which cause fat retention. What we asked ourselves was this: what happens to people when substances to which they are exposed are not dumped into fat? To answer this question we retraced our steps into toxicology textbooks. And here, in addition to what we were looking for, we also found some recognition of the protective role of fat. In their standard work, *Toxicology: The Basic Science of Poisons*, Casarett and Doull state: 'The toxicant while it is stored often does no harm to the organism. Storage depots should therefore be considered as protective organs . . .' The authors comment that there is a possibility of 'a sudden increase in concentration of chemicals in the blood should there occur a rapid mobilization of body fat', but they do not speculate on the possible consequences of such mobilization.

One extreme consequence was one of the clues we had at the

beginning of our PFR Syndrome search. Some years ago large numbers of migratory sea birds were found floating, dead, in the North Sea. The cause of death was a mystery for some time; eventually it was attributed to PCBs – polychlorobiphenyls, chemicals used in a great many industrial processes – although how they caused death was unclear. We now know what happened. Migratory birds put on fat to store energy for their long flights. During such flights a rapid mobilization of this body fat occurs, and any substances stored in it are released. These birds must have picked up lethal doses of PCBs, stored them protectively but incidentally in fat, and then released them with tragic consequences.

Fortunately for humans, our metabolisms are not so simple, nor are we as crucially dependant on cyclical use of fat reserves, so mobilization is not fatal. However, some consequences of uncontrolled mobilization and/or heavy toxic exposure, are already apparent in the medical literature, and there is suggestive evidence pointing to yet more.

Disease associated with poisoned fat can affect many systems of the body. Examples come from the effects of crash diets and unaccustomed strenuous exercise, both of which mobilize fat rapidly. From the other end, as it were, certain patterns of disease have become increasingly common in our chemically contaminated culture.

Of all methods of dieting, the very low calorie protein-based slimmers' drinks used to replace all meals are potentially the most harmful. Their success in rapidly metabolizing fat stores is also the source of their danger. There are various forms of such diets. According to a report of the Royal College of Physicians on obesity, in one year 'at least 60 deaths occurred in obese patients consuming liquid protein diets'. Of course, the true death toll due to these diets cannot be known and the real figure may be much higher.

The best documented result of rapid mobilization of fat is heart attack. Ironically, some people launch into drastic diet and exercise regimes in order to avoid heart attacks. The tragic outcome of their efforts results from a failure to recognize the nature of the problem. Controlled studies of very low calorie, high protein diets reveal that potentially fatal disturbances of heart rhythm develop quickly. You will now appreciate that, as the liver is directly connected to the heart, this is what may be expected. Whether from drastic diet/exercise regimes or low calorie, high protein diets, the result tends to be the same; a high and sometimes fatal loading on the heart.

The disruption of the body's systems for metabolizing stress hormones under conditions when liver glutathione stores are decreased will add to this problem. Very low calorie diets rapidly deplete the levels of this crucial detoxifying substance. Under these circumstances, stress hormones may build up to levels which damage the heart.

It is easy to see how the media, and many doctors, may periodically be persuaded to launch campaigns against the dangers of exercise. They rarely pick on diets. Unfortunately, their criticism is generally founded on a prejudice, which they hope will strike a sympathetic chord with their audience, rather than on any real understanding of what is happening in peoples' bodies. When it comes to the positive creation of health, their view is lamentably short-sighted.

This short-sightedness is typified by the debate on heart disease and dietary fat – the butter versus margarine controversy. Those who studied causal links between heart disease and diet discovered that a high consumption of saturated fats was associated with increased risk. What they failed to highlight was the fact that these are also the most heavily contaminated fats. Heart disease seems to be associated, not with fats as such, but with polluted fats – particularly processed fats. Cholesterol, contrary to popular belief, is harmless providing it is pure and natural. Other types of fat pollution have yet to be investigated, but we believe that risk to the heart and blood vessels is a feature of many types of contaminants of fats.

Males are more at risk of heart and circulatory disease than females. Hardening of the arteries, where cholesterol is deposited in atheromatous plaques in the blood vessels, seems to be a response of the male metabolism with its limited ability to generate toxic adipose tissue. Cholesterol plaques form in major blood vessels, but these are only dangerous when they degenerate and cause the walls of the blood vessel to ulcerate. We believe that this ulceration is caused by contaminants laid down in the plaque. There are cultures where the diet causes extensive lining of the arteries with cholesterol, but because of its purity it does not lead to the formation of degenerative plaques, or to heart disease.

Recent research has shown that the distribution of fat on the body is important in heart attacks. The person whose waist measurement is very large in relation to their hip size has a much higher risk of coronary episodes. This accumulation of belly fat is typical of the PFR Syndrome. Victims can be quite slim apart from a large deposit of fat around the waist; such uneven distribution is a feature of toxic adiposity. So this type of fat deposit, particularly among males, may lead us through toxic input and a limited ability to store in fat, to heart disease as a possible outcome. Heart and circulatory diseases are the most common cause of death in the world; it may be significant that women are not at such high risk until their hormone balance changes, becoming more like the male after menopause – as does their metabolism and body shape.

Another area of possible problems arises because the molecules stored in adipose deposits would be likely to have a high affinity for other fatty tissues in the body. Such tissues include the nervous system; nerve cells are largely composed of fat. Our brains are 60 per cent fat, mostly cholesterol. Clearly we should look for damage to the nervous system; the problem is that low-level disruption may be difficult to detect.

We would expect behaviour to be disrupted in a variety of ways, and while this may be easy to observe, it is difficult to link cause and effect in a definite way. However, studies of diet and delinquency have revealed just such a link. Other commentators have pointed to society-wide changes in behaviour, such as increased violence and decreasing literacy, and linked such phenomena to environmental chemical pollution. We do know one case where the circumstantial evidence appears convincing. Kathy suffers from multiple sclerosis, a disease of the fatty tissues which sheath nerves. She had always been plump, male friends considered her a model of buxom feminity, and a happy, lively person. She smoked and had three children, none of which influenced her very stable state. Kathy decided to go on a strict crash diet. Her aim was to shed forty pounds in three months to achieve her target weight. While on this diet she noticed no obvious ill-effects, apart from those associated with deliberate self-starvation such as loss of energy, hunger and sleeplessness. The day she decided to strip the varnish from an old sideboard is indelibly fixed in her memory. As she got to work with paint-stripping chemicals, waves of giddiness came over her. Before she could get away, she collapsed.

Now she relates the onset of multiple sclerosis to this episode. The combination of crash diet and exposure to a cocktail of chemicals sadly produced the sort of result we would predict. When Kathy recovered from her collapse, it was some weeks before she realized that something serious had happened to her. At first she did not recognize the symptoms; now, five years later, she does not ever expect to be free of multiple sclerosis.

This disease, along with heart disease, is characteristic of our culture. That is to say it is only found in significant numbers where the Western way of life has spread. Although neither disease has a simple single cause, both are associated with diets high in sugar and animal fats – precisely the type of diet which we would expect to produce the highest levels of toxic adiposity. The degeneration of the nervous system associated with this diet is, we believe, a consequence of chronic poisoning with fat-soluble toxins.

How many other diseases of the nervous system result from these ubiquitous hazards? It is of course impossible to say. Not only is there insufficient information to make a reasoned

estimate, the fact that our culture believes that all such substances are safe inhibits objective research into any diffused
effects of this sort.

In Britain two-thirds of the billion gallons of pesticides
sprayed each year are organophosphates. These chemicals are
related to nerve gases, yet through such widespread use,
including in domestic fly-killers, they are present in the air all
the time. The range of accepted symptoms associated with
chronic poisoning by this most popular insecticide includes the
following: anxiety, uneasiness, emotional instability, giddiness,
insomnia, drowsiness, tinnitus (noises, usually ringing, in the
ear), inability to get on with family and friends, depression and
weepiness.

These are precisely the symptoms that hundreds of thousands
of women suffer all the time in our society. It has been shown in
the United States that these symptoms can continue for years
after exposure to insecticides. These are also the complaints for
which tranquillizers are prescribed, perhaps to 10 per cent of
the population of the Western world. The cause of the
symptoms, and the means of their modification, provide good
business for many companies who make both products.

Could it be that we are witnessing nothing less than the
population-wide modification of behaviour and emotion by our
casual use of these substances? It is a theme which has been used
in science fiction, but is it really all that far from the truth? We
would not wish to imply that such an effect is intentional. And
we accept that those charged with regulating the use of such
substances may be genuine in their beliefs; but we are equally
sure that they are culturally blinkered to the exact nature of
such a catastrophe.

We must go on to consider possible problems associated with
changes in fatty tissues. These in turn include diseases linked
with female hormones, which are actually produced by fat cells.

The most frightening possible association is with cancer of
the breast. Like the other conditions we have mentioned, breast
cancer is much more common in developed countries, and it has

become increasingly common over the course of this century. Once more it is statistically associated with a diet high in animal fats, and is more common among fatter women. Certain drugs, notably oral contraceptives and the antihypertensive, reserpine, have also been linked with an increased susceptibility to breast cancer.

The female breast is an organ that is composed largely of fat. The focus of toxins in this fat is clearly indicated by the high level of poisonous residues found in mothers' breast milk, at times rendering it unfit for human consumption, an issue we shall return to later. Unlike most fatty parts of the body, the tissue of the breast is quite active; it undergoes marked changes with the monthly cycling of hormones.

We suspect that the metabolic activity of the natural monthly cycle could produce a situation where toxins stored in breast fat have been put there in error. The aim of storing them on a long-term basis is clearly thwarted by the action of the hormones. Their regular release could mean that they are more likely to trigger local cancers before they can be reabsorbed into fat in other sites.

Animal experiments with drugs and chemicals suggest a special sensitivity of mammary tissues to certain carcinogens. Those that are chemically related to natural female hormones, paradoxically, most often induce such cancers. For example, depo-provera, the controversial contraceptive injection, causes mammary tumours in beagle bitches.

The incidence of breast cancer has risen by more than 40 per cent over the past twenty years. Part of the reason for this is almost certainly our increasing consumption of synthetic hormones, not only in the Pill but also in residues in dairy produce and meat. The other toxic residues are likely to compound the problem. Because of the active nature of breast fat, even those with protective PFR are unlikely to escape. The only solution is to avoid accumulating toxic residues in your body.

Cervical cancer is also hormone-linked, and has also been

rising in incidence very rapidly over the past few decades. A direct link with the PFR mechanism is as yet unclear, but the association with smoking suggests that it may be triggered by toxic residues. The induction of the CP 450s and the subsequent production of reactive intermediaries may be the key factor. Other contributory elements could be oral contraceptives and poor diet.

Recent increases in skin cancer, associated with white skin exposed to unaccustomed sun, suggest another cancer possibility. Is the cancer, as is conventionally held, caused by the overexposure to ultra-violet radiation in strong sunlight, or is it more likely to be caused by the gallons of screening chemicals applied to the skin?

Recent concern has been focused on the cancer-generating effects of cyclical use of brown fat reserves. Brown fat is metabolically active fat, sited mainly on the back. It is mobilized by adrenalin to keep us warm under a variety of stresses. If we rely on brown fat for heat generation, its cyclical use could increase the risk of cancer from the release of its contaminants.

Various specialists have estimated that 80 per cent of the cancers we now suffer are environmental in origin. Cancer, more than any other condition, is what the body strives to avoid. We all produce faulty, potentially cancerous, cells all the time. In the normal course of events they are recycled by the liver as part of its normal activity. Cancer is helped to take hold if either the detoxification system is overloaded, or the production of cancer cells outstrips the clean-up capacity of the body. Very many of the pesticides and other chemicals discussed in this book not only overload detoxification systems, but have also been shown to be capable of causing cancer.

Typically, cancer victims lose weight, sometimes wasting away with horrifying rapidity. As they waste, they develop secondary tumours, frequently in the liver. At this point the toxic load is overwhelming all the body's coping mechanisms. Quite logically, there are many parallels between the innocent food diet necessary for escape from PFR and the Bristol Diet, which was developed as part of the gentle way of curing cancer.

We are convinced that following the PFR Escape Plan, and weaving its principle elements into your permanent way of life, will not only keep you slim, but also substantially diminish any risk you may run of developing cancer.

Many women put the health of their children before their own. Some implications of the PFR Syndrome are crucial for anyone who is thinking of having a baby.

During pregnancy all metabolic processes are more active. Fat stores are used by the mother's body to provide for the needs of the developing baby. This will be especially true if she is making efforts to avoid putting on too much weight during pregnancy. Throughout pregnancy the baby will be exposed to the toxins which are being mobilized from its mother's fat. Pesticide residues and other chemicals have been found in the placenta and in the blood of the umbilical cord; it is believed that the fetal liver is involved in the metabolism of these substances. It seems that nature, accepting the limited detoxification capacity of the mother's liver, couples the baby's liver up in tandem to share the work. There is a logic in this; if the mother were fatally poisoned, the baby would die as well, so they work together to avoid this possibility.

Under the loading of potential toxins the mother is subjected to, it is inevitable that her baby is exposed to these residues from its earliest moments of life. And with modern obstetric practices, the fetal liver is sometimes exposed to such a load of drugs that signs of malfunction are apparent at birth.

Neo-natal jaundice, once a relatively rare occurrence, reached epidemic proportions at the height of the popularity of birth induction. Even without induction, anaesthetics and pain-killers given to the mother will reach the baby across the placental wall, stressing its metabolism and developing detoxification systems.

Newborn babies can have a horrifying range of chemicals circulating in their bloodstream. One ten-month-old was recently found to have residues of eight pesticides in his blood, one of which was Dieldrin, supposedly banned in most Western countries. His doctor fears long-term damage to the baby's nervous system, including deafness. The doctor treating this baby stated, 'It is neither normal nor natural to have pesticides in the blood. A few years ago the high levels I deal with today would have been unthinkable.' Another member of the team treating the baby commented, 'Fruit and vegetables should carry a government health warning like cigarettes.'

After birth, and before the baby can develop any extra coping capacity, the toxic load can build up. Human babies need fat for normal development, and breast milk is 4 per cent fat. Unfortunately, this fat contains toxins which have been concentrated by the mother's body. If she has been exposed to high levels of pollution or has an inefficient detoxification system, she may be feeding her baby a concentrated dose of chemicals. All samples of human milk tested in recent years have been found to contain pesticides.

One recent research paper showed that the concentration of DDT and related compounds in breast milk can give babies a daily dose in excess of the maximum intake set by the World Health Organization. Babies whose mothers have been exposed to PCBs at work show rising blood levels of this pollutant. The chemical remains in the infant's body for several years.

Feeding your baby on cow's milk is not likely to improve the situation. Although cow's milk contains less DDT and other contaminants found in mother's milk, it has a contamination profile of its own. The cow's body concentrates the toxins to which it is subjected just as the mother's does; these will come from the chemically sprayed meadows, from the contaminated feedstuffs produced for cattle and from the increasing numbers of drugs routinely given to animals.

If this were not bad enough, people are actively exploring ways of feeding animals which can only add to the problem. Orville Schell's *Modern Meat, Antibiotics, Hormones and the Pharmaceutical Farm* details just how far this process has gone. Any feelings that we may have overstated the issue of contaminated food and its effects may be settled by reference to this book. Among many examples, such as the effect of premature puberty produced by overdosing chickens with growth hormones, Schell notes the activities of a waste reclamation company. They specialize in 'exotic feeds for beef and dairy cattle'. Among the products this company sells as cattle feed are cardboard, sawdust, ground bark, ground cardboard and grapefruit peel, and various grades of waste paper bringing with it glue, ink, clay and plastics. If we are prepared to treat our bodies as dustbins, why not the bodies of other animals?

Some years ago infantile eczema was more common among bottle-fed babies. Today the situation is reversed; breast-fed infants are more likely to suffer this unpleasant allergic condition. The reason is undoubtedly the increasing pollution level of mothers' milk.

The problems of PFR, and the risk of passing toxins on to your baby, can add a whole new and more realistic view to family planning. Many of the problems for children are avoidable – if you detoxify your body, its inputs and your personal environment before you conceive. The Plan has all you need. You should stick to YES foods as much as possible, and eat on Schedule 1 through your pregnancy and while you are breast feeding.

Vegetarian mothers have been shown to have lower residue levels in their milk. As a consequence, while they keep to a sensible, balanced diet that provides plenty of protein and other nutrients, their babies are healthier.

Hyperactive children present a problem for growing numbers of parents. While we would not go as far as some drug companies, who have a vested interest in describing most children as hyperactive, there is no doubt that it is a condition which afflicts many. It has been convincingly linked with additives in favourite foods, especially colouring and flavouring chemicals. If you have this problem, changing your family over to the detoxifying diet as you change your eating habits should help. The health and sociability of your children will improve and you will avoid the problem of childhood obesity. The addictive nature of many of these substances may make the change-over irksome; you just have to persevere.

Allergic children are often, as we would expect, born to PFR victims. Over the years there have been many television programmes on the problems of allergic and hyperactive children. We now recognize that the mothers, almost without exception, were those heavy, over-rounded types typical of the PFR Syndrome. Because their systems could not cope with its chemical loading, they had become fat. During pregnancy the overload was passed on to their babies, damaging their immune systems before birth.

The implications of the PFR Syndrome and its cause are widespread. It is likely that not only is every person on the planet to some degree poisoned, but that all of us suffer some adverse effect from these substances. It is illogical to demand more medical care in an environment of increasing hazards. If you are concerned with adopting healthy habits, you should not accept this situation.

The truth of our health problems is that we are at war. In every part of the environment we have created, humans are in retreat. While it is generally assumed that human activity, with all the benefits it brings, is a universal good, this is far from the truth.

You are suffering from a random effect of pollution. This pollution is not the old-fashioned sort that we have now largely cleaned up, the smoke and soot of crude industry; it is a new, more subtle and insidious enemy. Perhaps it is easiest to think of it as molecular terrorism. As with terrorists in a foreign land, you may not know which are the enemy, which will attack you or what you can do to defend yourself against the continual threat they pose.

Looking outside the boundaries of your home can be depressing. If you live near a chemical factory, or in the country where pesticides continually contaminate the air, your health will be at risk. Detoxifying your food may simply not be enough; you may have to start on the world.

We believe passionately that health should be the first priority of our social and economic systems. To the degree that it is not, and to the degree that these systems actually harm us, they must be judged as failures in meeting human needs. Not so long ago, those growers who insisted that organic was best were mocked. Advocates of the Soil Association message were dismissed as 'the muck and magic brigade'. More recently, many people thought groups such as Friends of the Earth, Greenpeace and even CND were composed of cranks and weirdos. At the same time people believed those who were telling them that DDT and nuclear radiation were safe. With the passing of time more people are realizing who was right and who was wrong.

This book, and its plan to help you lose weight caused by toxins in your environment, should not be necessary. That it is should make you angry. Angry enough to add your voice to those who are trying to change the world in which we live for the better. Addresses of organizations campaigning for conservation and environmental improvement can be found in Appendix 5.

The causes of the ill-effects on our health that we have been discussing are within our control. Political expediency and profit are the forces which generate the problems; inertia, habit and ignorance maintain them. The politics of food and environment are increasingly on the agenda in every country in the world; you have to help keep them there until rational answers are forthcoming. The profit motive is amenable to modification; if enough people stop buying contaminated rubbish to eat, sooner or later they will stop making it. Point your purse in the right direction every time you shop.

There is no other answer to the larger problem than to change the priorities of the major polluters of the world: industry and the agribusiness food producers. The same goes for government; people in government want power, they should only have it on terms of a real priority for human welfare.

In Britain we have a classic case of priority conflict; new water regulations have been introduced by the EEC, and Britain's water boards say they cannot comply with the standards –

indeed, one spokesperson was complaining about the cost burden of having to apply for so many exemptions! Britain's water is increasingly in doubt. What used to be a classic third world health problem now affects most countries; along with many parts of America, Britain cannot afford clean water. Yet the British government considers it reasonable to spend untold billions on the unusable virility symbol of a Trident submarine nuclear defence system.

More than twenty years ago Rachel Carson's *Silent Spring* sounded a warning which caught people's imagination. Since then the problem has gone underground; we have not learned the essential lesson of that warning. We should have understood that it was necessary to work towards a way of living that enhances life, rather than refining the process of widespread spraying of death. We need to change the philosophy that accepts such methods, so that organically grown food becomes the norm rather than a scarce commodity. That pure, unpolluted air, water and food should be available to everyone, not just those who search and travel miles to get them.

In the narrowest sense, we are dealing with products developed for profit by the multinational chemical corporations. While incidents such as Seveso and Bhopal give some insight into the potential danger of their activities, the claimed benefits for their products and activities usually outweigh reactions against such disasters, no matter how horrific.

Discussions on the activities of chemical companies generally centre around details of safety, either of process or of particular products, and of the employment they provide. In terms of human health such finely detailed assessment is not very helpful. The problem they pose is global; our response needs to be of a similar magnitude. We need to be able to make decisions in philosophical terms which will either allow and encourage their activities, with real safeguards and monitoring, or control and phase them out. To take such decisions we need to have a suitable perspective of what they are actually doing.

As the American cosmologist Carl Sagan so eloquently expressed it, both in his television series and book, *Cosmos*, we are star-stuff. All the living matter on our planet, including us, is made up from large molecules that could only have been assembled in the nuclear furnace of a failed star. The mass of unreacted atoms in our cosmos are just not complex enough to perform the very basic operations required both to evolve and sustain life.

The molecules on our planet which are involved in life have been cycling through a vast variety of forms ever since they first began to replicate in the primeval soup some 3,500 million years ago. The organic view of nature, and our food production from it, accepts and works with this reality. The aim of modern organic food producers is to enhance and strengthen the cycles of life.

Until very recently in human history everyone lived, and died, as an integral part of this cycle. Even our technology, based on refining and purifying basic material, did little to interfere. Its products were all biodegradable and could be reabsorbed into the broader cycle of the biology of the planet.

In the sixteenth century a French philosopher, Réné Descartes, produced a system of belief, Cartesian Dualism, which influences our attitudes and behaviour to this day. His system is commonly referred to as 'mechanistic philosophy'; it is rooted in the belief that our intellectual life is divorced from the actions of our bodies, which can be regarded as machines. We in our turn are divorced from the rest of creation by an assumption that our nature is special, an assumption which allows us to behave as if the rest of the world has been provided for us to treat as we will. After Descartes, many others erected complementary belief systems which had the net effect of confirming our unique position; we became progressively divorced from the rest of the biosphere and the reality of life itself.

The recent search for alternative answers and growing interest in holistic health are reactions against the implications and effects of mechanistic philosophy. Some would lay at its door blame for all the most profound and seemingly insoluble problems which now confront humanity.

The mechanistic belief system allows us to treat food species as products requiring processing in the most efficient way possible. The cruelty of factory farming, the infliction of suffering and distortion of basic animal needs, as well as the destructive mining of sterile fields with fertilizers and biocides, is simply a logical extension of such beliefs.

As indeed is the production of the artificial molecules, which not only sustain such agriculture, but increasingly sustain large numbers of us. The reality of the mechanistic philosophy is that, to a limited degree, it will deliver the goods. It is the limit of its ability to do so, and the cost of its accomplishment, that we are questioning.

What the chemical manufacturers are doing is picking up the remnants of an earlier life-cycle, and giving its molecules another chance at bio-activity. Most of the feed stock for the chemical industry comes from oil. Oil is the remains of untold billions of small life forms which existed millions of years ago. Their remains have been trapped in the earth's strata, and stabilized. Coal is the rough vegetable equivalent of this process, and its by-products can also form chemical raw materials.

The carbon atoms and other products in these deposits are part of the planet's stock of star-stuff. In the past these molecules were activated and enlivened by the sun in exactly the same way that we and the other life-forms alive with us are today. Instead of their remains being recycled directly in the life chain, they were lost and became locked up. Until recently, our only use for them was to burn them to release the stored energy.

Industrial chemistry changed that wasteful process. Chemists found that they could attach an almost unlimited number of other substances on to the obligingly cohesive carbon atoms, and thus create a theoretically infinite number of new, entirely artificial substances. The process is referred to as molecular roulette; substances are produced, what they will be is not known. A new molecule may be a dye, a drug, a food, a solvent, a poison, or have any one of a thousand possible uses.

Some of the products will be very bio-specific, such as the DDT molecule which seems to be highly motivated to become part of living matter once more. The effects of a growing number of the products of the industrial chemist are causing increasing concern. The problem is that it takes time to recognize the dangers. DDT was declared safe in the past, when those who should have known better were blinded by its possibilities and commercial potential. How many of today's chemicals will be seen as dangerous in a decade or so?

Products fall into two crucial categories: those which are biodegradable, and those which are not. Biodegradable substances are eventually broken down, usually by bacteria, and their components are made available for uptake by other life-forms. There is little to criticize in this; but what of the vast number of manufactured substances which are not biodegradable? Again these fall into two categories: those which are inert and those which are bio-active.

It is this latter class which causes harm. Many such substances are either designed to enter our food, or do so by chance. Others are released into the environment and make their own way into bio-processes and the food chains. Some we apply so that they may enter directly into our bodies. Once we set up chains of pollution in this way it is very difficult to eliminate them.

Why do we need to make philosophical choices about such problems? The answer is because our philosophy directs our culture, and our culture produces our beliefs. The attitudes we adopt to practical, everyday issues are based in their turn on these beliefs.

It is our philosophy which allows the nuclear industry to turn the Irish sea into a radioactive hazard. Everywhere we look in our man-made environment there are problems of pollution of growing magnitude. The Club of Rome's computer model of world dynamics consistently indicates that it is pollution which will finally destroy us, rather than nuclear or other short-term holocausts. Your PFR problem is a direct experience of the process they are pointing towards.

Unless we act as a species, as you have had to act as an individual, we will overload the capacity of our planet to recover. Just as you have experienced the effects of personal overload to your detoxification system, so the entire planetary biosphere could confront the same problem. The degree to which it could recover is a matter of great debate. Mechanists basically believe that there is no problem; they have a tradition of holding on to this belief until forced by disaster to modify their view. Holistic philosophers, and their varied Green allies, believe that the world is finite, and its capacities are similarly finite. Until we know for sure where the limits of that finality are, caution would be advisable, prudence commendable and a total rethink desirable.

References

Abbott, D. C., *et al.*, 'Organochlorine pesticide residues in human fat in the United Kingdom 1976–7,' *British Medical Journal* (November 1981) 1425–28.

Adam, K. and Oswald, I., 'Sleep helps healing,' *British Medical Journal*, (November 1984) 1400–01.

'Wholefoods may give you more than you bargained for,' Soil Association *Quarterly Review* (Winter 1982–3) 7–8.

Nutrition Reviews, 43 (February 1985).

ARC/MRC Committee, Food and Nutrition Research. (HMSO, 1974) 160–172.

Arenillas, L., 'Amitriptyline and body-weight,' *The Lancet*, (February 1964) 432–3.

Beller, A. S., *Fat and Thin*. (Farrar, Straus & Giroux, 1977).

Bird, A. G., 'Allergic reactions during anaesthesia,' *Adverse Drug Reaction Bulletin* (February 1985) 408–11.

Bourne, W. R. P., 'Seabirds and Pollution.' R. Johnson (ed.) *Marine Pollution* (Academic Press).

Bray, G. A., 'Definition, measurement and classification of the syndromes of obesity,' *Int. J. Obesity*, 2 (1978) 99–112.

British Medical Association & Pharmaceutical Society of Great Britain, *British National Formulary* (The Pharmaceutical Press, 1984).

Byrivers, P., *Goodbye to Arthritis*. (Century, 1985).

Cannon, G. and Einzig, H., *Dieting Makes You Fat*. (Sphere, 1984).

Consumers' Association, 'E-numbers, doctors and patients: food for thought,' *Drug & Therapeutics Bulletin*, 22, no.11 (1984) 41–2.

Dahlgren, B. E., 'Hepatic and renal effects of low concentrations of methoxyflurane in delivery ward personnel,' *J. Occ. Med.*, 22 (1980) 817–9.

Denning, J., 'The hazards of women's work,' *New Scientist* (January 1985) 12–15.

Denning, J., *Women's Work and Health Hazards: A Bibliography* (TUC/London School Hygiene and Tropical Medicine 1984).

Doull, J. *et al.* (eds.), Casarett and Doull's *Toxicology, the Basic Science of Poisons* (Macmillan, 1980).

Erlichman, J., 'Good enough to eat?' *New Health* (June 1985) 28–33.

Eyton, A., *The F-Plan Diet* (Penguin, 1982).

Forbes, A., *The Bristol Diet* (Century, 1984).

Fritsch, A. (ed.), Center for Science in the Public Interest, *The Household Pollutants Guide* (Anchor Books, 1978).

Garner, D. *et al.*, 'Cultural expectations of thinness in women,' *Psychological Reports*, 47 (1980) 483–91.

Gear, A., *The Organic Food Guide* (Henry Doubleday Research Association, 1983).

Gillman, A. G. *et al* (Eds.): *Goodman & Gillman's The Pharmaceutical Basis of Therapeutics* (6th edition, Macmillan 1980) Chapter 1.

Goulding, R., 'Chemical hazards in the home and workplace,' *Practitioner*, 227 (1983) 1363–9.

Grant, E., *The Bitter Pill: How Safe is the 'Perfect Contraceptive'?* (Elm Tree Books, 1985).

Hanssen, M., *E for Additives* (Thorsons, 1984).

Hildyard, N., *Cover Up: The Facts They Don't Want You to Know* (New English Library, 1981).

Kendler, K. S., 'Amitriptyline-induced obesity in anorexia nervosa: a case report,' *Am. J. Psychiat.* (1978) 135, 1107–8.

Kenton, L. and Kenton, S., *Raw Energy* (Century, 1985).

Lappe, F. M., *Diet for a Small Planet* (Ballantine, 1982).

Laseter, J. L., 'Body burden and sources of toxic volatile organics,' paper given to the McCarrison Society Conference (1984).

Lawrence, F., 'Additives anonymous,' *New Health* (April 1985) 30–5.

Lee, D. H. K. (ed.), *Handbook of Physiology*, section 9: 'Reactions to environmental agents' (American Physiological Society, 1977).

Mackarness, R, *Not all in the Mind* (Pan, 1976).

Mackarness, R., *Chemical Victims* (Pan, 1980).

MAFF, *Household Food Consumption and Expenditure* 1982 (HMSO, 1984).

Melville, A. and Johnson, C., *Cured to Death: the effects of prescription drugs* (Secker & Warburg, 1982).

Millstone, E., 'Food additives: a technology out of control?' *New Scientist* (October 1984) 20–4.

Morley, J. E. and Levine, A. S., 'The central control of appetite,' *The Lancet* (February 1983) 398–401.

Morse, D. L. *et al.*, 'Cut flowers: a potential pesticide hazard.' *Am. J. Pub. Health*, 69 (1979) 53–6.

Murray, A. J. and Portmann, J. E., *Aquatic Environment Monitoring Report*, no.10. (MAFF Directorate of Fisheries Research, 1984).

Nakra, B. R. S. *et al.*, 'Amitriptyline and weight gain: a biochemical and endocrinological study,' *Curr. Med. Res. Opin.* (1977) 4, 602–6.

Nicolson, R. S., *Association of Public Analysts Surveys of Pesticide Residues in Food, 1983, J. Assoc. Publ. Analysts*, 22 (1984) 51–7.

Paykel, E. S. *et al.*, 'Amitriptyline, weight gain and carbohydrate craving: a side effect,' *Brit. J. Psychiat.* (1973) 123, 501–7.

Paul, A. A. & Southgate, D. A. T., McCance & Widdowson's *The Composition of Foods*, (HMSO, 1978).

Polishuk, Z. W., 'Effects of pregnancy on storage of organochlorine pesticides,' *Arch. Environ. Health*, 20 (1970) 215–7.

Rose, C., 'Pesticides: the first incidents report,' Friends of the Earth (1984).

Royal College of Physicians, 'Obesity.' *J. Roy. Coll. Phys.* (January 1983).

Royal College of Physicians & British Nutrition Foundation, 'Food intolerance and food aversion,' *J. Roy. Coll. Phys.* 18, no.2 (1984) 83–123.

Ruckpaul, K. (ed.), *Cytochrome P-450* (Academic-Verlag, 1984).

Schauss, A., *Diet, Crime and Delinquency* (Parker House, 1981).

Schell, O., *Modern meat: antibiotics, hormones, and the pharmaceutical farm* (Random House, 1984).

Stellman, J. M. & Daum, S. M., *Work is dangerous to your health* (Vintage Books, 1973).

Sterling, *et al.*, 'Building illness in the white-collar workplace,' *Int. J. Health Serv.*, 13 (1983) 277–87.

Waldbott, G. C., *Health effects of environmental pollutants* (C. V. Mosby, 1973).

Watts, J., *An investigation into the use and effects of pesticides in the UK* (Friends of the Earth, 1985).

Wolff, M. S., 'Occupationally derived chemicals in breast milk,' *Am. J. Ind. Med.*, 4 (1983) 259–81.

World Health Organization, *Pesticide Residue Series*, Nos. 1–5. (World Health Organization, 1972–6).

Recommended Reading

Bull, David, *A Growing Problem: Pesticides and the Third World Poor* (Oxfam, 1982).

Cannon, G. and Einzig, H., *Dieting Makes You Fat* (Century, 1983).

Gear, A. (ed.), *The Organic Food Guide* (The Henry Doubleday Research Association, 1983).

Gibson, S., Templeton, L. and Gibson, R., *Cook Yourself a Favour, Help Yourself to Better Health* (Johnston Green Publishing Group, 1983).

Hills, Lawrence, *Organic Gardening* (Harmondsworth: Penguin Books, 1977).

Kenton, L. and S., *Raw Energy* and *Raw Energy Recipes* (Century, 1984).

Lappe, F. M., *Diet for a Small Planet* (Ballantine Books, 1982).

Mackarness, R., *Chemical Victims* and *Not all in the Mind* (Pan, 1976 and 1980).

Melville, A. and Johnson, C., *Cured to Death* (Secker and Warburg, 1982).

Orbach, S., *Fat is a Feminist Issue* (Hamlyn, 1979).

Physical Fitness, exercise plans developed by the Royal Canadian Air Force (Penguin Books, 1964).

APPENDIX 1

'E' Codes

The material in this Appendix comes from 'Look again at the label – chemical additives in food', a special report by the Soil Association prepared by Peter Mansfield.

Colourings

	BEWARE **AZO DYES**	**SUSPECT**	**SAFE**
E100			E100 Turmeric
E101			E101 Vitamin B2
E102	E102 Tartrazine		
E104	E104 Quinoline Yellow		
107	107 Yellow 2G		
E110	E110 Sunset Yellow		
E120		E120 Cochineal[3]	
E122	E122 Carmoisine, Azorubine		
E123	E123 Amaranth		
E124	E124 Ponceau 4R		
E127	E127 Erythrocine		
128	128 Red 2G		
E131	E131 Patent Blue V		
E132	E132 Indigo Carmine		
133	133 Brilliant Blue		
E140			E140 Chlorophyll
E141			E141 Chlorophyll
E142	E142 Green S, Lissamine Green		
E150		E150 Caramel[2]	
E151	E151 Black PN		
E153			E153 Carbon
154	154 Brown FK		
155	155 Brown HT		

BEWARE	SUSPECT	SAFE
E160		E160 Relatives of Vit.A
E161		E161 Relatives of Vit.A
E162		E162 Relatives of Vit.A
E163		E163 Anthocyanins
E170		E170 Chalk
E171		E171 Titanium Oxide
E172		E172 Iron Oxides
E173	E173 Aluminium	
E174	E174 Silver	
E175	E175 Gold	
E180 E180 Pigment Rubine		

NOTES

(1) Azo Dyes — Dangerous to asthmatics, hyperactive children, those sensitive to aspirin.

(2) Caramel — Prepared by various processes, some of which may incur vitamin B6 deficiency. The definition is being simplified. 98% by weight of all the colouring used in foods.

(3) Cochineal — Can cause hyperactivity in children.

Preservatives

BEWARE	SUSPECT	SAFE
E200		E200 Sorbates[1]
E201		E201 Sorbates[1]
E202		E202 Sorbates[1]
E203		E203 Sorbates[1]
E210	E210 Benzoates[2]	
E211	E211 Benzoates[2]	
E212	E212 Benzoates[2]	
E213	E213 Benzoates[2]	
E214	E214 Complex Benzoates[2]	
E215	E215 Complex Benzoates[2]	
E216	E216 Complex Benzoates[2]	
E217	E217 Complex Benzoates[2]	

BEWARE		SUSPECT	SAFE
E218	E218 Complex Benzoates[2]		
E219	E219 Complex Benzoates[2]		
E220	E220 Sulphur Dioxide[3]		
E221	E221 Sulphites		
E222	E222 Sulphites		
E223	E223 Sulphites		
E224	E224 Sulphites		
E226	E226 Sulphites		
E227	E227 Sulphites		
E230	E230 Biphenyl[4]		
E231	E231 Biphenyl[4]		
E232	E232 Biphenyl[4]		
E233			E233 On citrus and
E234			234 banana skins
E236		E236 Fomic acid[21]	
E237		E237 Formate[21]	
E238		E238 Formate[21]	
E239	E239 Hexamine[9]		
E249	E249 Nitrite[8]		
E250	E250 Nitrite[8]		
E251	E251 Nitrite[8]		
E252	E252 Nitrate[8]		
E260			E260 Acetic acid
E261			E261 Acetates
E262			E262 Acetates
E263			E263 Acetates
E270		E270 Lactic Acid[5]	
E280			E280 Propionates[6]
E281			E281 Propionates[6]
E282			E282 Propionates[6]
E283			E283 Propionates[6]
E290		E290 Carbon Dioxide[7]	
E296			E296
E297			E297

NOTES

(1) E200-203 Sorbic Acid — From mountain ash berries.

(2) E210-219 Benzoates — Dangerous to allergics, asthmatics, hypersensitives.

(3) E220-227 Sulphur Dioxide etc. — Beware on uncooked raw fruit. Dangerous to asthmatics, hypersensitives. Lowers Vitamin E content of flour. Lowers Vitamin B1 content of various foods.

(4) E230-232 Biphenyls — Beware on citrus peel.
Some probably penetrates to the flesh.

(5) E270 Lactic Acid — Beware in food for very small babies.

(6) E280-283 Propionates — Migraine sufferers may do well to avoid these.

(7) E290 Carbon Dioxide — Enhances absorption in stomach.
Increases effect of alcohol.

(8) E249-252 Nitrite, Nitrate — Highly controversial. May combine with amines in the stomach, producing highly cancer-forming nitrosamines. Interacts dangerously with the blood cells of infants.

(9) E239 Hexamine — May upset intestines, urinary system, or less often the skin. Possibly cancer forming.

Anti-Oxidants, Emulsifiers, Stabilisers, Miscellaneous

BEWARE	SUSPECT	SAFE
E300		E300 Ascorbates
E301		E301 Ascorbates
E302		E302 Ascorbates
E304		E304 Ascorbates
E306		E306 Vitamin E
E307		E307 Vitamin E
E308		E308 Vitamin E
E309		E309 Vitamin E
E310	E310 Gallates[1]	
E311	E311 Gallates[1]	
E312	E312 Gallates[1]	
E320	E320 BHA[22]	
E321	E321 BHT[22]	
E322		E322 Lecithins
E325	E325 Lactates[2]	
E326	E326 Lactates[2]	
E327	E327 Lactates[2]	
E330		E330 Citrates
E331		E331 Citrates
E332		E332 Citrates

BEWARE	SUSPECT	SAFE
E333		E333 Citrates
E334		E334 Tartrates
E335		E335 Tartrates
E336		E336 Tartrates
E337		E337 Tartrates
E338		E338 Phosphates
E339		E339 Phosphates
E340		E340 Phosphates
E341		E341 Phosphates
350		350 Malates
351		351 Malates
352		352 Malates
353		353 Metatartaric Acid
355		355 Adipic Acid
363		363 Succinic Acid
370	370 Heptonolactone	
375		375 Vitamin B
380		380 Citrates
381		381 Citrates
E385	E385 Salt of EDTA[3]	
E400		E400 Alginates (seaweed)
E401		E401 Alginates (seaweed)
E402		E402 Alginates (seaweed)
E403		E403 Alginates (seaweed)
E404		E404 Alginates (seaweed)
E405		E405 Alginates (seaweed)
E406		E406 Agar
E407	E407 Carrageenan[4]	
E410		E410 Natural Gums
E412		E412 Natural Gums
E413		E413 Natural Gums
E414	E414 Acacia Gum[5]	
E415		E415 Natural Gums
E416		E416 Natural Gums
E420		E420 Sorbitol
E421	E421 Mannitol[6]	
E422		E422 Glycerol
430	430 Stearates[7]	
431	431 Stearates[7]	
432	432 Polyoxyethylene[8]	
433	433 Polyoxyethylene[8]	
434	434 Polyoxyethylene[8]	
435	435 Polyoxyethylene[8]	
436	436 Polyoxyethylene[8]	

BEWARE	SUSPECT	SAFE
E440		E440 Pectin
442	442 Ammonium phosphatides	
E450	E450 Polyphosphates[9]	
E460		E460 Cellulose
E461		E461 Cellulose
E463		E463 Cellulose
E464		E464 Cellulose
E465		E465 Cellulose
E466		E466 Cellulose
E470	E470 Fats, soaps[20]	
E471	E471 Fats, soaps[20]	
E472	E472 Fats, soaps[20]	
E473	E473 Fats, soaps[20]	
E474	E474 Fats, soaps[20]	
E475	E475 Fats, soaps[20]	
E476	E476 Fats, soaps[20]	
E477	E477 Fats, soaps[20]	
E478	E478 Fats, soaps[20]	
E481	E481 Fatty Acids	
E482	E482 Fatty Acids	
E483	E483 Fatty Acids	
491	491 Sorbitans[10]	
492	492 Sorbitans[10]	
493	493 Sorbitans[10]	
494	494 Sorbitans[10]	
495	495 Sorbitans[10]	
500		500 Carbonates
501		501 Carbonates
502		502 Carbonates
503		503 Carbonates
504		504 Carbonates
507	507 Chlorides[11]	
508	508 Chlorides[11]	
509	509 Chlorides[11]	
510	510 Chlorides[11]	
513	513 Sulphuric Acid[12]	
514	514 Sodium Sulphate	
515		515 Potassium Sulphate
516		516 Calcium Sulphate
518		518 Magnesium Sulphate
524	524 Caustic Soda[12]	
525	525 Caustic Potash[12]	
526		526 Calcium Hydroxide
527	527 Ammonium Hydroxide[12]	
528		528 Magnesium Hydroxide

BEWARE	SUSPECT	SAFE
529	529 Quick Lime	
530	530 Magnesium Oxide	
535 535 Ferrocyanides[13]		
536 536 Ferrocyanides[13]		
541 541 Phosphate[14]		
542	542 Bone Phosphate[15]	
544 544 Polyphosphates[9]		
545 545 Polyphosphates[9]		551 Silicates
551		552 Silicates
552		553 Talc
553		
554 554 Silicates[14]		
556 556 Silicates[14]		
558	558 Bentonite	559 Kaolin
559		570 Stearate
570		572 Stearate
572		
575	575 Glucono delta Lactone	576 Gluconates
576		577 Gluconates
577		578 Gluconates
578		

FLAVOUR ENHANCERS[16]

620	620 Glutamic Acid	
621	621 Monosodium Glutamate	
622	622 Other Glutamates	
623	623 Other Glutamates	
627	627 Guanylate[17]	
631	631 Inosinate[17]	
635	635 Guanylate and Inosinate[17]	
636	636 Maltol 'fresh bake' flavour[16]	
637	637 Ethyl Maltol – sweetener[16]	
900		900 Dimethicone
901		
903		901 Bees Wax
904		903 Carnauba Wax
905	905 Mineral Hydrocarbons[18]	904 Shellac
907		907 Wax
920		920 Amino-acid derivative
924	924 Bromate[19]	
925	925 Chlorine[19]	
927	927 Azoformamide[21]	

NOTES

(1) Gallates — A benzoate, not permitted in foods intended for young children. May harm asthmatics, those sensitive to aspirin, hyperactive children.

(2) Lactates — To be avoided for very young children.

(3) EDTA — May disrupt absorption of Iron, Zinc and Copper.

(4) Carrageenan — Irish moss, a seaweed; may however cause ulcerative colitis, and may decompose to a carcinogen. Worst in drinks.

(5) Acacia Gum — Known to be toxic at 100%; some confections get to 45%!

(6) Mannitol — Occasionally produces hypersensitivity.

(7) Stearates — May produce skin allergies; a possible cause of kidney stones.

(8) Polyoxyethylenes — Very little information available; may alter absorption of fat.

(9) Polyphosphates — Used to retain moisture in meat products, they can easily be abused to inflate the weight (and price) of a product, though this is an offence in Britain. Beware particularly of chicken and ham.

(10) Sorbitan esters — Very little information available. May increase gut absorption of paraffins, which are irritant.

(11) Chlorides — Several are capable of corrosive effects on the intestine, and perhaps disturbances of body fluids. Very little information available.

(12) Acids & Alkalis — These are all corrosive, in sufficient quantity. Little information is available as to how they are used.

(13) Ferrocyanides — We depend for our safety on nothing disturbing their low absorption from the intestine.

(14) Contains Aluminium — Suspected to be capable of harm in some people.

(15) Bone phosphate — Vegetarians would wish to avoid this.

(16) Flavour enhancers — Make the food taste better than it really is. Along with salt and sugar, largely responsible for distorting appetites and encouraging over-eating. Almost certainly implicated in the epidemic of obesity in young people.

(17) Purines — Prohibited from foods intended for young children. Gout sufferers, and rheumatics generally, should avoid these.

(18) Hydrocarbons — That is liquid paraffins, which as cathartics may cause anal seepage and soreness, and stool looseness, in some people.

(19) Bleaches	Doubts exist about safety. In flour, destroys Vitamin E and other nutrients. Capable of major intestinal upset, and convulsions.
(20) Fats, soaps	Little information is given. Could in quantity interfere with intestinal function and absorption.
(21) Formates	Formic acid very irritant to skin. All have diuretic effects (on the kidneys).
(22) BHA, BHT	Currently subjects of intensive safety research, because of many doubts. Either may contribute indirectly to wastage of body stores of Vitamin D, or cause hyperactivity. Neither permitted in foods intended for young children.

A full copy of this report may be obtained from the Soil Association, 86 Colston Street, Bristol BS1 5BB.

Prescription Drugs which May Cause Weight Gain

This list cannot be exhaustive for two reasons. First, new drugs are being introduced into the market continually and therefore the list will not be up to date; second, drugs that are capable of inducing weight gain in a minority of people may not yet be known to do so – especially if they cause weight loss in some individuals and gain in others. This is a common pattern with allergic reactions, and many liver-related drug reactions are believed to be associated with allergy.

Drugs named on this list will not cause weight gain in all those who take them. Side-effects of drugs are almost always a product of a unique interaction between the nature of the substance and the individual metabolism of the person who takes them. Therefore any drug you take or have been taking should be regarded as one of the possible causes of your PFR problem.

These lists have been compiled from standard reference sources (*Martindale: The Extra Pharmacopaeia* and *British National Formulary*). These sources give side-effects for whole classes of drugs and we acknowledge that weight gain may not have been specifically related to all brands listed here. However, since data on weight changes with each particular product may not be available, while side-effects of one member of a drug class are likely to be shared by others in the same class, we have endeavoured to include similar forms.

Group 1 Hormones

Generic drug names: clomiphene citrate, danazol, progesterone, dimethisterone, dydrogestrone, oestradiol, estropipate, ethinyloestradiol, ethisterone, ethynodiol diacetate, flumedronone acetate, fosfestrol sodium, gestronol hexanoate, hexoestrol, hydroxyprogesterone hexanoate, lynoestrenol, medrogestone, medroxyprogesterone acetate, megestrol acetate, mestrenol, methallenoestril, noresthisterone, norethyrodrel, levonorgestrol, oestradiol, oestriol, promethoestrol dipropionate, quinestrol, quingestanol, stilboestrol. Branded products which include these drugs are listed below.

Oral contraceptives (the contraceptive Pill): all types.

The Pill can induce a variety of changes in liver function. One important effect is to slow down the action of one of the main detoxifying enzymes, aryl hydrocarbon hydroxylase, which deals with substances such as petrochemicals, by as much as a third. Slow liver function has been demonstrated in overweight women taking the Pill. Abnormal liver function associated with the Pill has been related to severe allergic reactions to foods and chemicals. Recovery after discontinuing Pill use is often slow, but Evening Primrose Oil is helpful.

Contraceptive injections

Medroxyprogesterone acetate   Depo-Provera

Preparations used for hormone replacement therapy and menstrual problems

Ethinyloestradiol
Oestradiol   Benztrone, Hormonin, Progynova
Oestriol   Ovestin
Conjugated oestrogens Premarin
Piperazine oestrone   Harmogen

Quinestradol	Pentovis
Danazol	Danol
Progesterone	Cyclogest, Gestone
Dydrogesterone	Duphaston
Ethisterone	Gestone-oral
Hydroxyprogesterone hexanoate	
	Proluton Depot
Medroxyprogesterone acetate	
	Depo-Provera, Provera
Norethisterone	Primolut N, Utovlan
	Cyclo-Progynova, Menophase
	Mixogen
	Prempak, Trisequens
	Controvlar, Norlestrin, Ovran
	Ovranette
	Controvlar, Norlestrin

Male sex hormones and antagonists

Cyproterone acetate	Androcur
Mesterolone	Pro-Viron
Methyltestosterone	Plex-Hormone, Virormone-Oral
Testosterone	Testoral Sublings
Testosterone esters	Primoteston Depot, Restandol
	Sustanon
	Virormone

Other hormones

Clomiphene citrate	Clomid, Serophene

Group 2 Drugs for diabetes

Insulin: any form when dose exceeds requirements

Tolbutamide	Pramidex, Rastinon
Chlorpropamide	Diabenese, Melitase

Glibenclamide	Daonil, Euglucon
Acetohexamide	Dimelor
Glibornuride	Glutril
Gliclazide	Diamicron
Glipizide	Glibenese, Minodiab
Gliquidone	Glurenorm
Tolazamide	Tolanase
Glymidine	Gondafon

Group 3 Drugs acting on the central nervous system

Antidepressants

Amitriptyline	Domical, Elavil, Lentizol, Saroten Tryptizol, Limbitrol, Triptafen
Butriptyline	Evadyne
Clomipramine	Anafranil
Desipramine	Pertofran
Dothiepin	Prothiaden
Doxepin	Sinequan
Imipramine	Praminil, Tofranil
Iprindole	Prondol
Lofepramine	Gamanil
Maprotiline	Ludiomil
Mianserin	Bolvidon, Norval
Nortriptyline	Allegron, Aventyl, Motipress, Motival
Protriptyline	Concordin
Trazodone	Molipaxin
Trimipramine	Surmontil
Phenelzine	Nardil
Iproniazid	Marsilid
Isocarboxazid	Marplan
Trancypromine	Parnate, Parstelin

Tranquillizers and drugs used for schizophrenia and other psychoses
(some of these drugs may also be prescribed for nausea, vertigo,
Menieres Disease and other problems.)

Chlorpromazine	Largactil, Chloractil, Dozine
Clopenthixol	Clopixol
Fluphenazine	Moditen
Fluspirilene	Redeptin
Lithium carbonate	Camcolit, Liskonum, Phasal, Priadel
Lithium citrate	Litarex
Methotrimeprazine	Nozinan, Veractil
Oxypertine	Integrin
Pericyazine	Neulactil
Perphenazine	Fentazin
Pimozide	Orap
Pipothiazine	Piportil
Prochlorperazine	Stemetil, Vertigon
Promazine	Sparine
Sulpiride	Dolmatil
Thiethylperazine	Torecan
Thioridazine	Melleril
Trifluoperazine	Stelazine

Other generic types associated with weight gain include:
acetophenazine, butaperazine, carphenazine,
chlorproethazine, chlorprothixene, clomacrom phosphate,
cyamemazine, dixyrazine, fluopromazine, loxapine,
mesordazine benzenesulphate, molindone, oxaflumazine,
pecazine, penfluridol, pipamazine, piperacetazine,
prothipendyl, spiclomazine, sulforidazine, sultopride,
thioproperazine, thiothixene.

Group 4 Drugs for prevention of migraine

(see also beta-blockers, below)

Methysergide	Deseril
Pizotifen	Sanomigran

Group 5 Drugs for heart disease and high blood pressure

Beta-blockers

Most drugs of this type, including forms not listed here, are known to precipitate 'weight changes'. This list includes those which are associated with weight gain.

Acebutol	Sectral, Secadrex
Atenolol	Tenormin, Tenoret
Metoprolol	Betaloc, Co-Betaloc, Lopresor, Lopresoretic
Nadolol	Corgard, Corgaretic
Oxprenolol	Apsolox, Laracor, Slow-Pren, Slow-Trasicor, Trasicor, Trasidrex
Penbutolol	Lasipressin
Pindolol	Visken, Viskaldrix
Practolol	Eraldin
Propranolol	Angilol, Apsolol, Bedranol, Berkolol, Inderal, Inderetic, Inderex
Sotalol	Beta-Cardone, Sotacor, Sotazide, Tolerzide
Timolol	Betim, Blocadren, Moducren, Prestim

Other drugs prescribed for high blood pressure

Clonidine	Catapres, Dixarit
Minoxidil	Loniten

Pargyline   Eutonyl
Reserpine, rauwolfia alkaloids
                         Abicol, Decaserpyl, Enduronyl,
                         Harmonyl, Hypercal, Rautrax,
                         Rauwiloid, Serpasil

Cholesterol reducing drugs

Clofibrate   Atromid-S

Group 6 Anti-inflammatory drugs

Indomethacin   Artracin, Imbrilon, Indocid, Indoflex,
                         Indolar, Mobilan, Rheumacin LA
Sulindac   Clinoril

Group 7 Antihistamines

Astemizole   Hismanal
Cyproheptadine   Periactin

APPENDIX 3

Organic Food Suppliers

Importers and Producers of Organic Food

These companies are primarily wholesalers, but they will be able to give you the name of your nearest retail shop. Some also sell direct to the public.

Harmony Foods, Adelphi Works, Cobbold Road, London NE10
Tel: 01 451 3111.

Organic Farms & Growers (OFG) Ltd., 9 Station Approach, Needham Market, Ipswich, Suffolk IP6 8AT
Tel: 0449 720838.

Organic Farm Foods, Unit 7, Ellerslie Square, Lyham Road, London SW2
Tel: 01 274 0234.

Infinity Foods Ltd., 25 North Road, Brighton, BN1 1YA
Tel: 0273 690116.

Höfels Pure Foods, Stowmarket Road, Woolpit, Suffolk
Tel: 0359 40592.

Johanus (UK) Ltd., William Morris Yard, Forest Row, East Sussex, RH18 5NW
Tel: 034 282 4588.

Bristol Organic Farm Foods Ltd., Unit 2, Albert Crescent, St Phillips, Bristol
Tel: 0272 712015.

Wholefood, 24 and 31 Paddington Street, London W1
Tel: 01 486 1390 and 01 935 3924.

Brand names of foods which are generally organic

(but check the labels – some of these companies also market food which is not grown by organic methods).

Doves Farm, Hofels, Infinity, Neal's Yard, Pimhill, Prewetts, Harmony, Springhill

Retail suppliers of organic foods

Very few of these shops sell exclusively organic foods. Ask the staff or check labels. This list includes only some suppliers – there are many more.

Cranks Health Food Shop, 8 Marshall Street, London W1
Also other branches.

Neal's Yard Wholefood Warehouse, 21 Shorts Gardens; also Farm Shop, Dairy, Bakery, etc: Neal's Yard, Shorts Gardens, Covent Garden, London WC2.

Wholefood of Baker Street, 24 Paddington St, London W1.

Safeway, supermarkets in London and the South. Organic produce is marked with a special label.

Infinity Foods, 25 North Road, Brighton.

Southern Health Foods, Wellington Centre, Victoria Road, Aldershot.

Arjuna, 12 Mill Road, Cambridge.

Rainbow Wholefoods, 16 Dove Street, Norwich.

Spa Health Foods, 60 The Mall, Clifton, Bristol.

The Granary Traditional Foods, 15d Causeway Head, Penzance.

York Wholefood, 98 Micklegate, York.

The Circle Health Food Centre, 311 Dickson Road, Blackpool.

Wholemeal, 158 Queen's Road, Leicester.

Real Foods, 37 Broughton Street, Edinburgh.

Roots and Fruits, 457 Great Western Road, Glasgow.

Basic Movement

This routine is for those whose range of movement and ability may be severely restricted.

The object is to encourage you to extend your range of movement by progressively increasing the use of muscle groups you might normally ignore. You should not try to do too much at any one time – for you little but often is the key. Be cautious, if you are very overweight; straining and immobilizing yourself through over-exertion is the last thing you want to do. Gradual steady progress is what you are after. As you become more mobile you will be able to put more effort in, which in turn will increase your mobility. You will have created a positive cycle which will lead you to success.

Try to do all the movements listed below, but if you can't, don't worry – just do as many as you can for now. You will see that we do not say how many times or how long you should continue each movement for. You must judge this; at the outset you should stop as soon as you feel the effort, once you have been through the routine a few times you will learn how much you can manage. Do as much as you can; if you continue while you are enjoying it that is the best guide. Sooner or later this routine will seem too easy or too boring. Then it has served its purpose and you are ready to move on to something else!

Preparation: For you this may be as demanding as a four hour workout is for Daley Thompson, so make sure you are ready. A relaxed and positive state of mind is essential; perhaps some meditation and breathing may be helpful. Wear clothing that is comfortable and will not hinder your movement. Make sure nothing will interrupt or distract you. Have some soft and easy music on if you feel it will help.

1) With your feet flat on the floor, stand with your back against a wall. Stretch up and push as much of you against the wall as you can – paying particular attention to getting your shoulders up and back. Once you are in your best position, hold it, and relax and breathe as deeply and slowly as you can. Concentrate on filling yourself up with as much air as you can get in, and let it out slowly. Really feel your chest rise and expand with each breath. Don't worry if your heart knocks a bit or you feel a touch of giddiness – that is just the effect of the load coming off, or the extra oxygen. Keep breathing deeply as long as it feels good, but do at least six really deep and slow ones. While you are in this position search for the feeling in your back and shoulders. Try to locate the feeling so that being upright with your shoulders back becomes your normal way of standing.

2) Away from the wall, stand comfortably, with your feet a foot or so apart and your arms loose at your sides. Now just bend your knees a little so that you sink down a few inches – you must judge how far you can manage – then swing your hands up to your shoulders, and reach up as far as you can above your head. As you stretch your arms upwards, straighten your legs again, and push up on your toes to reach even higher. Keep your arms straight and lower them to your sides, and go down from your toes. Finally bend your knees again, and repeat. Breathe in as you go up and out as you come down. Move at an easy pace and try to make it smooth and continuous, don't jerk. Raise and lower your arms both in front and to the sides to add a little variety. Feel what is happening to the parts of you that are moving. You could break this into two movements if necessary, by sitting and doing the arm movement and stretch up, and then standing and doing the leg movement, using the back of a chair for balance if necessary.

3) Either seated or standing, as you did the previous movement, reach your arms out straight at the sides at shoulder height. Stretch out as far as you can with your finger tips. Now slowly move your straight arms so that your finger tips go round in small circles. Breathe in as they go up and back, out as they go forward and down. Once you have got the rhythm right, make the circles as big as you can. Keep your back straight and the movement slow and easy, take the timing from your breathing. You may prefer to start by just letting your arms dangle at your sides and shrugging your shoulders into circles. Breathe the same way if you do this.

4) Everyone needs a chair for this one. Stand behind the chair so you can use the back as a support. The movement you are aiming for is to bend forward from the waist, with your legs straight, so that your back becomes parallel with the floor like an ironing board. You may not be able to do that at the beginning, so just bend forward as far as you can, then straighten up, using your hands on the chairback as necessary. Concentrate on keeping your back straight throughout. Breathe out, bending forward and in when you straighten up. Slow and easy, once more. Don't go too far at first.

5) Lie on your back. A firm surface with a rug is best. Arms by your sides, feet a little apart. One leg at a time, bring your knee up until your thigh is pointing straight up. Don't try to keep your leg straight, just let your foot dangle. Then lower your knee and straighten out your leg. Repeat for both legs, breathing out as you raise your knee and in as you lower it. Later on you could try swinging your foot up to straighten your leg once your thigh is vertical.

6) Same position. Stretch your arms out above your head, with arms straight so that you point to the ceiling. Then lower them back behind your head. Breathe out as you raise and in as you lower. For variety you can do the same movement to the sides instead of above your head. Or you could begin by stretching your arms out to the sides, and bending

them up first at the elbow, then pushing up towards the ceiling. Have a few relaxing deep breaths while you are lying on your back. Then when you are ready, complete your session by getting up and going for a walk. You should aim for steady continuous movement, slowly if necessary. Shoulders back (remember the wall feeling), swing your arms, loose and smooth. Don't worry about how far or fast, just enjoy the sensation of movement. Afterwards have a treat; perhaps a bath or shower.

As you become more active you will increase the range of movement you can manage. This routine allows for that. When doing 2) you could end up doing full squats, and then leaping in the air. 4) could have you touching your toes, and 5) could turn into leg raises energetic enough for the flattest tummy.

But for now concentrate on enjoying moving. Do a session whenever you feel like it during the day. As you do more, you will discover that it has a positive reinforcing effect; at first you should do it when you feel good, but soon you will discover that being active when you do not feel good will actually change your state; it will make you feel better. Once you make this dis-covery, you have taken the first step in achieving real control over your body and self.

When you are ready to move on to something else, start thinking about dance. It can provide energetic and enjoyable movement for the whole body – and you just have to do it.

Dance

We want you to think about dance as one of the oldest forms of human recreation (re-creation). Dance has always fulfilled a variety of needs: self-expression, relaxation, transcendence, communication, and a number of other emotional needs. Our mundane world limits this advantageous activity mainly to the young. This is wrong. All ages need to regain the innate abilities of dance.

Do not believe you are: too old, too fat, too awkward or too ugly. None of that is important. You may be self-conscious, most of us are. But dance can turn and twist that into something more valuable: consciousness of self.

There are two routes to dance. One is to become totally conscious of every part of your body, to direct each movement and posture and timing; this is the method of the professional dancer. The other is to feel every part of your being; to evolve movement as a partnership between the facets of your self, let your body influence its own direction with your mind as the means.

Take the feeling route. Try to let movement slide into you, using music as the stimulus. Movement should pervade and persuade you, take you along. Let go. Let it take you wherever it will! It may be a soft, sensuous experience or a driving physical expression of feeling.

Dance can regenerate the very core of your being. Because it is a self-directed activity, it will involve many levels of being, both physical and mental, in creating feedback loops. These can build up sensations and energy, becoming almost frighteningly exhilarating, or just a gentle exploration of part of your self. Either way, the ancient rhythms will help you unlock and grow.

How do you do it?

To begin with, you will start with simple conscious movements to suitable music, copying the way you've seen others move. Think of all the dance from cultures around the world: maybe you incline towards the African sometimes? Or is there a little of the stamping Aborigine about you? Don't let yourself be limited by our society's assumptions about dance.

You may find it easier if you watch yourself in a large mirror – but not if the mirror puts you off! You may want to introduce some of the jogging/jumping movements you do as exercise. Fine. While you are moving, try to relax enough to let your body take over. The music should help. Listen to it, let your body go.

Think carefully when you choose your dancing music. You

should select something that speaks to you personally, that communicates directly with your being. It could be anything from a Beethoven quartet to the Rolling Stones; it could be punk or romantic, or even disco dancing music. The crucial thing is that it moves you, and you move with it.

Don't be disheartened if nothing magical happens. Enjoy the music and the movement, and sooner or later it will.

Dance as long and as often as you like, alone or in company. See if you can get a partner to join in sometimes. But remember, you are dancing for yourself.

Organizations working towards an unpolluted world

Action on Smoking and Health, 27–35 Mortimer Street, London W1N 7RJ Tel: 01 637 9843.

Compassion in World Farming, 20 Lavant Street, Petersfield, Hants. Tel: 0730 64208.

Friends of the Earth, 377 City Road, London EC1 Tel: 01 837 0731. Also many local branches.

The McCarrison Society (for medical and other professionals concerned about nutrition). Secretary: Mrs Margaret Clark, 36 Bowness Avenue, Oxford OX3 0AL Tel: 0865 61272.

Soil Association, 86 Colston Street, Bristol BS1 5BB Tel: 0272 290661.

The Ecology Party. Ask at your library for your local contact.

Greenpeace, 36 Graham Street, London N1 8LL.

The Schumacher Society. Contact via *Resurgence* magazine (available from 'alternative' and radical bookshops).

The Henry Doubleday Research Association (an international body of organic gardeners with a strong research orientation), Covent Lane, Bocking, Braintree, Essex CM7 6RW.

The Good Gardeners' Association (an international association of organic gardeners), Arkley Manor, Barnet.

International Federation of Organic Agricultural Movements (an organization of groups and individuals with the common aim of encouraging sustainable agricultural methods worldwide). Secretariat: Gunnar Videgaard, Le Maioun, F84 410 Bedoin, France. English-language bulletin from The Organic Gardening Research Centre (Rodale Press), Box 323, Kutztown, Pennsylvania 19530, USA.

APPENDIX 6

Further help

This book is intended to enable you to safely loose your persistent fat, cellulite or troublesome flab. We want you to succeed in that objective.

The method described in the Plan is based upon our experience in assisting clients of Life Profile with the same problems – we know that it works. However, because of the wide variability produced by individual differences, lifestyle and circumstances, some readers may have specific difficulties, or reach a sticking point which is peculiar to them. To help in these cases we have produced a special programme within the Life Profile system which is available to readers of this book.

If you would like to take advantage of this, this is what you should do:

1) Write a summary of the action you have so far taken in following the Plan. Note particular difficulties you have experienced, and also the successes you have had.

2) Give a basic personal outline. We need the following: your age, sex, brief medical and natal history, occupation, slimming and weight history. Additionally, we would like you to outline a typical day in your life, and tell us your likes and dislikes, your loves and hates.

3) If you have any thoughts or feelings about a particular difficulty, let us know.

Write to us at the following address:

Life Profile Ltd.,
37b New Cavendish Street
London W1.

Index

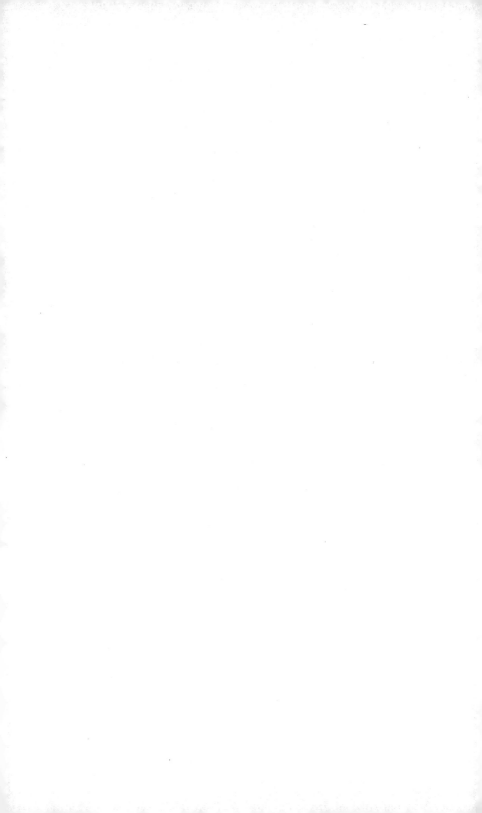

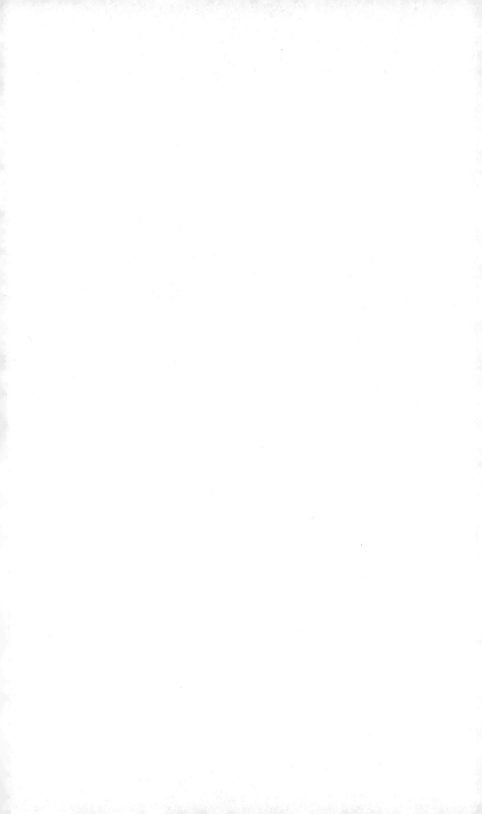